Aromat

A guide to their use in magick,

healing and perfumery

By
Ray Sherwin

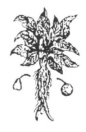

Also by Ray Sherwin

The Book of Results, first published by Morton Press in 1978, currently published by Baphomet Publishing in soft and hard back. Available through Amazon.

The Theatre of Magick, first published in 1981, currently published by Baphomet Publishing. Available through Amazon.

The Cardinal Rites of Chaos, Edition limited to 500 copies, published by Sut Anubis.

The Works of Aleister Crowley (Volume 1), Liber Agape, De Arte Magica. Ray wrote the introduction and annotated the text. Kadath Press 1986.

The Singing Tadpole; audio cassette and booklet, issued to friends in 1987.

The End of the World; a CD by Ray Sherwin and Nigel Mulaney, performing as "Best Before" 1997.

Contents

Illustrations

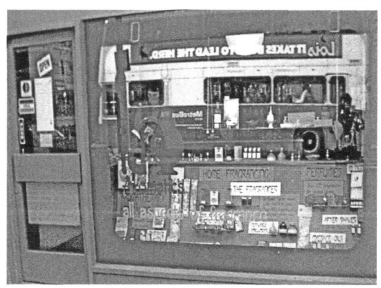

Above
Exterior of the shop in Boar Lane, Leeds. Unfortunately, the reflected bus mars any detail that there might have been in this 1983 snapshot.

Below
Shop interior 1984.

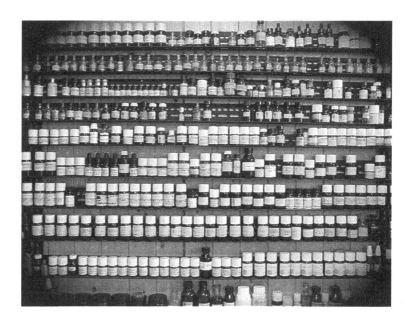

Introduction

I was born in Bradford in 1952. I have a little comment to make about that. I think of the fifties as a decade in black and white. The only odours lodged deeply in my memory are of the bread my mother used to make, the vanilla she used for baking, and the all pervading, foul stench of wool scouring, the first stage in the industry which brought fabulous wealth to a few Bradfordians and impenetrable fogs and smoke-blackened buildings to all of them.

Despite my parents' best efforts, there wasn't much magick about either. The best times of all were when we got away to the Yorkshire Dales. For a week or two my monochrome world gave way to glorious colour. The air smelled of nothing and the milk tasted of the herbs which the cows had been grazing on.

A passion for aromatics has been a part of my life for most of my adult life. That's what this book is about. However, my debut job was helping to run and build an inner-city adventure playground. That was the best job I ever had, but it didn't last forever.

After that I worked for the Scientology organisation for a year, editing a magazine whose name I can no longer remember. In the late sixties and early seventies, Scientology was taking a thrashing from the British government and, of course, anything that government doesn't like has to be worth taking a look at. I found a few interesting things but nothing any worse than I'd seen in Christianity and Islam. Indeed, judging by results I would say that Scientology is considerably more benign.

Then I ran a photographic laboratory for a year or so. I still have an interest although these days I prefer digital. It's quicker, less messy and I'm not exposing my eyes and lung tissue to aggressive chemicals.

At the age of twenty-four I started Morton Press, a one man publishing company named after the village in Yorkshire where I still live with my family. Three years and fifteen published books later I was getting so thin I put my blue pencil aside and got myself a proper job.

For a couple of years I taught English and Theology in upper school. Then I did a year teaching at a local college. In the meantime I'd fallen in love with Egypt and determined to spend some time there. I upped and offed and was very fortunate to be offered a job at The Sadat Academy, the business studies department of Cairo University. There I taught undergraduates, journalists and a group of sinister individuals who worked for an un-named government ministry.

I was out of Britain for about eighteen months. On my way back I picked up a copy of the *Guardian* in Tel Aviv only to find that Margaret Thatcher had just cut thousands of academic jobs. It seemed like déjà vu. Thatcher had been Minister for Education while I was a student and had cut thousands of jobs then!

Back in Morton I was kicking my heels when, one brilliantly sunny afternoon I ran into my old chess adversary, Michael Hurst, at the village gala. He was demonstrating, but not flying, a hang-glider (his passion) to a group of slack-jawed village kids. It had been a couple of years since I'd seen him so I invited him round for a couple of beers.

I'm not sure why, but while we were catching up with each other I got out my impressive collection of essential oil samples. Michael's enthusiasm fired up immediately. "We could make a business out of this", reports his initial comment more or less verbatim. I wasn't at all sure but, nevertheless, we spent all our spare time from that evening scouting for decent premises in which we could try out our retail ideas. Suffice it to say, for now, that this was where my career in aromatics really began.

At the time of writing I've come full circle. I enjoyed my incursion into the world of food, but I've been tempted back into doing some product development and selling the odd bottle of patchouli to people who call in.

1

... A Bottle Of Patchouli...

"...where the dripping patchouli was more than scent – it was the sun!" *(From the album* Ambient Dub 2, *track 'Soma Holiday' by G.O.L.)*

By 1982 I'd developed a stock answer to a question I was being irritated by nine or ten times a week. Standing in my shop in Leeds, people would often, accompanied by a flourish of the hand to indicate the commodities surrounding them, ask me "How did you get into all this?"

At the time it must have seemed an unusual shop. Along with my slightly dozing, (it would be unfair to say *sleeping*) partner Michael Hurst, I'd taken the risk of setting up an aromatics shop on one of the famous streets in Leeds centre. We concentrated on essential oils and absolutes but, underneath our logo ran the legend 'All aspects of fragrance' and, true to our word, we also traded in aromatic herbs, incenses, joss sticks, fragrant candles and the enigmatic oil evaporators whose use had to be carefully explained to every single customer.

Nowadays most people have an idea of what oil evaporators and essential oils are. In the early eighties most of my friends thought I was quite mad to attempt to make a business out of selling substances and items that virtually no-one had ever heard of.

I dare say that, for the early eighties, Id Aromatics, (which we sold in 1990), was the strangest shop in town. There certainly wasn't anywhere else you could obtain mandrake root, oakmoss resin or dragon's blood powder and, looking around the shop, which was a veritable Aladin's Cave of strange liquids, powders and gruesome looking roots, I had no difficulty in sympathising with the folk who, rather aggravatingly, repeated the question "How did you get into all this?"

If I'd been totally honest, my answer to the question would probably have been "I haven't the foggiest idea", but that wouldn't have been very interesting or entertaining so I eventually developed the answer "I think it probably all started with a bottle of patchouli in the 1960s."

This answer worked quite well. Oil of *pogestomon patchouli* was widely known, often by the corrupted names *patch*, *petunia* or, worse, *hippy juice*. It was probably, with the exception of eucalyptus oil, the only essential oil that was widely recognised. In the 1960s I'd been seduced by patchouli oil which I bought from an Asian man in Bradford's John Street Market. He would carefully decant the precious fluid from an aluminium flask into a 10ml brown bottle and it was as much this process as the oil itself which prompted me to find out what kind of a substance this really was.

I discovered that it was an essential oil and then had to find out what that was. From there it took the work of a mere afternoon in the vaults of the library to reveal that patchouli was not the only essential oil – deep joy, there were thousands of them! The problem was that I couldn't lay my hands on any of them! Nevertheless, I had the patchouli and that's where my story begins.

The chances are that you've never come across a recipe that requires the inclusion of graveyard dust. At the time when we opened Id Aromatics there was, also in Leeds, a dodgy occult supply business whose owner used to collect dust from graveyards to be sure that one or two of his incenses followed the old recipes exactly. He could have saved himself the trouble (and the indignity!) if he'd known that graveyard dust was an old alternative name for powdered patchouli leaves.

I never found much use for patchouli leaves. The odour is less than pleasant and I suspect that most of the long-haired folk who bought the wretched stuff from me sold it on to their friends as cannabis leaf, a trick they probably wouldn't get away with these days.

The oil had come into pre-eminence in the 1960s because it was virtually the only substance powerful enough to deodorize bikers' leather 'originals'. Without going into the unpleasant details let's just say that 'originals' are disgustingly dirty leather or denim clothes whose odour might be likened to that of neglected toilets.

Afghan coat wearers also found refuge in patchouli oil. Pleasant to look at those hairy fringed coats might have been but their wearers were avoided as centres of pestilence if they'd ever been caught out in the rain. The instant it gets wet an Afghan coat begins to emit the miasma of rancid yak and, since the coats were not cheap, people were reluctant to jettison them just because of the smell.

Enter patchouli oil. (In his marvellous novel *Jitterbug Perfume*, Tom Robbins has his hero searching for a fragrance to cover, or at least to pleasantly modify the horribly caproic odour profile of the Great God Pan. Mr Robbins reports that even patchouli was not up to it and the remainder of the book concerns the exploit of developing and making a perfume that would do the job. Needless to say, a natural deodorizer stronger than patchouli exists only in myth and novel!).

There was yet another reason for the use of patchouli in the sixties. Many misinformed individuals thought that it obscured the smell of cannabis smoke. Occasionally one or two policemen would call into the shop and ask for a sniff at the patchouli. They were even more badly informed than the public and thought that patchouli and cannabis smelled identical! All these things added up to a popularity and notoriety that no other essential oil had enjoyed during the twentieth century. That popularity, however, was not without precedent.

The nineteenth century saw an even greater interest in

patchouli oil and for much less nefarious reasons (depending on your point of view). Expensive Kashmir shawls became the vogue in the 1860s. As with all desirable and expensive items it wasn't long before the copycats got to work and, by all accounts, very good forgeries started to be made – so good that only experts could tell by eye which shawls were genuine and which were not. I say 'by eye' advisedly because even people who were not experts could tell the McCoy from the ringer by its smell.

The Kashmiri shawls had a distinctive, musty aroma which the copies did not. It transpired that the genuine shawls were packed with patchouli leaves, perhaps because this was a cheap form of packaging at that time or, more likely, because the patchouli leaves helped to preserve the delicate, hand-loomed material from the ravages of insects. Once the counterfeiters realised this it didn't take them long to ship in the patchouli oil with which they could make their illusion complete and, as a result, patchouli began to enjoy a wave of popularity even greater than the one it experienced in the 1960s.

During my first visit to India in 1989, I lavished about £50.00 on a genuine Kashmir shawl, handmade from the finest raw material and signed by the weaver. It seemed enormously expensive at the time but shawls of this nature can no longer be bought outside Kashmir. The garment, which is about six feet by four can be pulled through the ring I wear on my fourth finger without effort or rolled up and kept in a pocket, yet it traps enough heat to boil an egg if the egg is wrapped in the shawl and the shawl held in the hands.

Reputations are forged when a commodity of great mystery becomes popular. It was said of patchouli, for example, that it was an aphrodisiac. At the time when I was running the shop it was my habit to offer clients a drop on the wrist if they expressed an interest in a particular oil.

One dark evening, just before closing time, an attractive woman walked in and asked for patchouli. I didn't offer her the usual sample because there was something about this individual that I knew would be almost overwhelmingly attractive if she put even a small amount on her wrist. I sold her a bottle of the oil and got rid of her as quickly as possible. I don't have the faintest recollection what the woman was like but the sensation of her appearance accompanied by the *imagined* smell of patchouli remains with me almost twenty years later.

Quite a long time afterwards I came across the research of Professor Torii at Toho University in Japan. The bottom line of his research into patchouli was that it has a direct effect on the action of the sympathetic nervous system. While this doesn't necessarily scream 'aphrodisiac!' it does indicate that some cases of impotence or frigidity might be assisted by the use of this oil. The sympathetic nervous system is adversely affected by stress which decreases libido. If the SNS is relieved from stress by the action of patchouli it is not impossible that libido might be increased.

For this and other, more empirical reasons, I tend to advise patchouli as part of a de-stressing regime. If it weren't for the weird reputation that patchouli acquired during the 1960s,

I'm reasonably convinced that it would now be one of the most important oils used in aromatherapy. As things stand it tends to be sidelined as 'just patchouli'.

The late Robert Graves, in my opinion one of the great classical scholars of the twentieth century, appears to have been of the opinion that patchouli was available as an oil at the beginning of the present era. In his *Claudius the God*, he includes the following cameo.

"Presently he (Herod) came down smelling very strongly of a peculiar oriental scent called patchouli, which was a standing joke at the palace: it was supposed to have an irresistible effect on Cypros (his wife). Caligula, whenever he smelled it on Herod, used to sniff loudly and say " Herod, you uxorious old man! How well you advertise your marital secrets!"

I'm not so convinced that it was available but it is possible that strong infusions of patchouli in oil (such as olive) were imported into Rome from India. Because they didn't have soap, the Romans relied on steam and oil to get their bodies clean.

In the mid-eighties a strange young man whom I called Strawberry, because he pestered the life out of me to get strawberry oil for him, confessed to me that he'd consumed a full 10ml bottle of patchouli oil. Naturally I asked him why, and it turned out that he'd overheard me talking to a client about taking oils internally (which I wouldn't recommend under normal circumstances). Nevertheless, Strawberry took it into his head and drank the bottleful. At the time it didn't seem to have any adverse effects but I most recently saw him

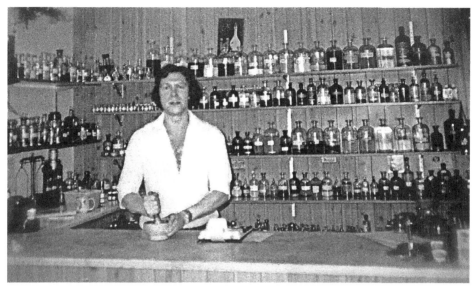

Above
Shop interior 1984, with Ray making a (very tiny!) batch of incense.

Below
Interior of the shop in Boar Lane in 1984. In the foreground is a pile of *Formaos* magazines. *Formaos* specialised in looking at the work and legacy of Austin Osman Spare.

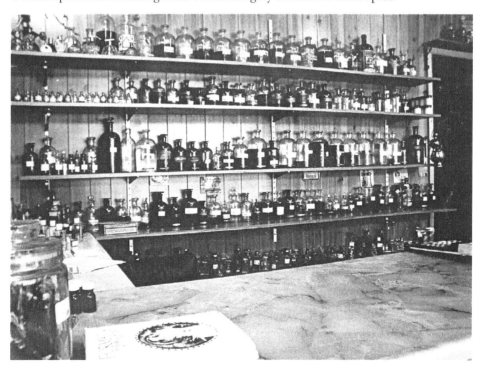

on television in the late nineties where he was being interviewed about his profession – he'd become a burglar, one of the clever ones who'd never been caught.

In view of this anecdote it seems reasonably safe to assume that patchouli oil is quite safe to use, especially if normal safety data is observed! My own observation about patchouli oil is that it heals wounds very quickly, probably because it contains *patchoulene*, a component similar to the famous *azulene* contained in chamomile oils (Roman and German). On the occasions when I've needed to use it, it appears to have formed a skin over the wound in double quick time and the wounds have always healed without going septic and without subsequent scarring.

It's difficult to be sure about some things in therapies, especially when you're relying on experience, but I strongly suspect that patchouli may be very useful in the treatment of impetigo and other unpleasant infections. As you'd expect, an oil which has a beneficial action on wounds is very useful in the treatment of certain types of eczema, especially where the skin is open and cracked.

As a first aid treatment for small wounds patchouli can be used undiluted. In treating larger areas a standard 3% dilution is more appropriate. Dilute it in coconut oil which contains a high proportion of lauric acid (see Chapter: The Fats of Life).

Whether the subject is wine, food or essential oils, we all have our personal preferences. I prefer Indonesian patchouli to all others and wouldn't use the oil at all if I could only get the

Chinese material. Methods of extraction differ from source to source. In Indonesia the herb is partially dried before being steam distilled. (I suspect the Chinese of urinating on theirs before doing anything else with it). It takes about a day to process 240 kilos of the dried herb, the yield of oil being in the region of 4%.

Good patchouli oil finds many uses. In perfumery it is used as a fixative to slow down evaporation and make the perfume last longer on the skin. It is particularly used in heavy, oriental type perfumes but also to an extent in rose bouquets along with clary sage. If one thinks of perfumes in terms of an organ with light notes at the top of the keyboard (eg sweet orange oil), patchouli is the penultimate key going downwards with only vetivert beneath it. It is therefore classified as a base note.

This is an extremely useful way of thinking for a perfumer but, in my opinion, has no benefit whatsoever in aromatherapy. If I want to cure myself of something I don't give a damn what the medicine smells like and, thinking about it, we all appear to have been brought up with the notion that the worse the medicine tastes, the more good it's likely to do us.

I'm verging on an appeal to forget the New-Age nonsense of treatments with carefully balanced top, middle and base notes. It's difficult enough to perform that balancing act by itself without also looking to include a healing function. The next time someone mentions synergistic blends or quintessential oils I might just be tempted to be less than polite. It's best to keep things as straightforward as possible and essential oils are immensely complex chemical packages even before we start to blend them together.

Despite the current vogue for oils straight from the still, my own preference is to age the patchouli oil by three or four years before selling it. In my view this gives a better product for both perfumery and for aromatherapy.

Aged or otherwise, patchouli is on the list of legally acceptable additives to tobacco and finds extensive use in this deplorable industry. If you like the smell of hand-rolling tobacco direct from the packet it's probably the inclusion of patchouli oil that makes such a deadly product smell so appetising.

I was once approached by 'an aromatherapist' who said he was happy to buy books from me but not essential oils. (I didn't sell books!) When I asked him why, he commented that our oils were not pure. He knew this because he'd done a stain test. This dubious test requires that a small amount of oil be put on a smelling paper or blotter, left to dry and then examined to see if there is any dry residue.

While this test is vaguely useful if one is forced to make an organoleptic assessment, one does have to know which oils one can successfully evaluate in this way. Patchouli, which is the one and only oil the 'aromatherapist' had stain tested is not one of the oils that can be evaluated in this way. It leaves an unmistakable stain.

Decoloured patchouli oil is available. This is produced largely for the soap industry since dirty-brown-looking soap has never been a market leader! However, the whole oil (the raw oil, if I might put it that way) should be used in aromatherapy and this applies to all the oils I can call to mind with the exception of camphor (use the white fraction only) and some of the fruit oils which are safer to use if the furocoumarins (eg *bergaptene*) have been removed. Patchouli oil is, generally speaking, a lighter colour than formerly because the Indonesian distillers are replacing their old iron stills with stainless steel equipment. The odour remains dark!

2

Hocus Pocus*

In Prehistoric (Neolithic) North Africa there lived, amongst many other people, a tribe of nomadic goat-herders. Recent archaeology suggests that they may have lived in or near the savannah which flourished at that time in the area now known as the Western Desert. Occasionally, these people noticed that their goats acquired a blackish, sticky substance on their fleeces and eventually they realised that if this substance were removed and burned, it provided a very fragrant smoke.

---

hocus pocus is a corruption of the words in the Catholic Mass *hic corpus meus* - this is my body. At one time it was used by lampooners and children's entertainers. These days it gets used to refer to activities on the dark side of normal or to mock New-Agers.

As a brief aside it is worth mentioning that the use of aromatic materials as incense is the origin of perfumery and of aromatherapy. The word perfume itself comes from the Latin words *per fumum*, meaning *through smoke*.

Having lived in North Africa, not far from the Nile delta, I can appreciate what kind of impact a pleasant smell had on the people who lived there at that time. Even living with the benefits of hot water and soap one starts to smell like a cheese one or two hours after a shower. In summer the coolest time of day is in the middle of the night. Even then, with all windows open and movement restricted as near as possible to nil, the perspiration pours off as if one were in a sauna.

The value of a fragrant substance was apparent to our nomads and they isolated the origin of the black sticky stuff. The goats 'collected' it as they grazed among the rock roses (labdanum). It can't have been long before the goats were removed from the equation. The invention of the *ladanesterion*, a flail with leather thongs later named after the plant by the Greeks, may have been the first technology to be related to aromatics. With it the nomads could flail the plants, the resin sticking to the thongs. From these it could be more conveniently squeeged off than it could from goats' fleeces. (They actually used sand to separate the labdanum from the ladanesterion, the sand being easily removed later).

Naturally enough, the labdanum resin so collected was much in demand and the nomads eventually gave up goat herding to become labdanum traders. They were so successful in this that they became the First Dynasty of Egypt. If you examine pictures of Pharaohs or of Osiris (the imagery is largely interchangeable) you will see that the arms are crossed over the chest, one hand bearing a crook (a legacy of the goat-herding days), the other hand bearing a flail (ladanesterion). The Pharaoh wears a false beard (even if female!) actually made from goat hair which was evidently stuck to the chin using labdanum.

The image of Jesus bearing a crook probably has more to do with the expression of his earthly power rather than the notion of the 'good shepherd'. Osiris, the previous bearer of the crook and also a dying and resurrected God, was the power, not only behind the Pharaonic throne but also the power behind the land of Egypt, being expressive of its fecundity. The imagery surrounding labdanum from pre-dynastic times has been in constant use ever since.

The importance of aromatics in Antiquity is thrown into sharp relief when it is realized that the humble rock rose is responsible for the iconic imagery so well known to us five thousand years later even if we have largely forgotten that the roots of this imagery are in incense (*per fumum*).

The oleo-resin is obtained from various species of *cistus*, principally *cistus ladaniferus*, the best material being collected between May and July. It was Dioscorides who first mentioned the ladanesterion method of collection but the first written mention of labdanum as a modern medicine occurred in 1589 when it was listed in *Dispensatorium Noricum*. Its use as a medicine does seem to stretch back into Antiquity though, because, although its principal uses were in incense and in the mummification process (along with the much better known frankincense and myrrh) there are ancient references to its use for liver and stomach problems as well as a remedy for breathing difficulties and for the loss of the hair.

The essential oil (which is very difficult to obtain commercially) has a specific gravity of 0.925 and its boiling point can be as high as 280 degrees, one of the reasons why it is an excellent fixative. Another reason is that, in the right proportion, it imparts an ambergris* note which is invaluable in some types of fine fragrances and lavender compounds.

While labdanum may have been the first aromatic commodity to be traded it seems reasonably self-evident that other materials would have been known in Antiquity. Thuja (Gr) refers to the various cedarwoods of North Africa and the Levant. It means 'to fumigate' or 'to sacrifice' which indicates that the Greeks valued cedarwood chippings as an incense. The notions of incense and sacrifice were closely linked in the mind of the Ancients, the smoke carrying the supplications of priests and others to the heavens.

The word 'fumigate' comes from the Latin *fumare* - to smoke and is the basis of our word perfume. The etymology of words connected with the subject of smell is a tangled trail always leading us back to man's first experience in controlling the nature of his olfactory environment - incense. That first experience probably happened at the same time as the discovery of fire since, in the case of labdanum, cedar, sandal, pine and many others, all man had to do was to throw it on the fire.

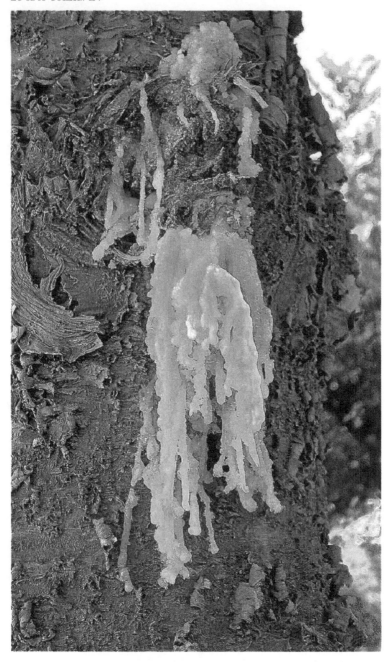

Pine resin almost spurting from the trunk of the tree.

In the early 1980s I was well aware that I was working at the end of a tradition which stretched back further than I cared to estimate. I expected that our shop would be visited by people with a requirement for incense but I wasn't in any way prepared for the variety of people or the variety of backgrounds from which they came. I made about forty 'standard' incenses for burning on charcoal and was happy to make bespoke incenses but until it started to happen I would never have anticipated that my personal interest might lead to having a witch-doctor and the vicar of the parish church standing at my counter happily discussing with each other what they did with the products that they bought from me. (I made chrism oil for the vicar. Only very occasionally did Christians ask me to make incense. Standard Church incenses are usually based on frankincense and benzoin and don't require any specialist knowledge. Making sure that they're producing smoke at the right time is another matter. This reasonably specialised technique is known as *thurify* and the person who does it is called the *thurifer*).

In fact, by the late eighties we supplied a good number of witch-doctors whose work took them all over Europe. One of them, doing very well to judge by his brand new, top-of-the-range Mercedes, was arrested right outside the shop by a WPC. It turned out that she'd berated him for parking there (quite right) but had arrested him for frightening her. I'm not making this up. Michael, my partner went to court to speak up for the man. The WPC had been frightened, she said, because when she'd asked him his occupation, he'd replied that he was a witch-doctor. Michael told the court that it was only reasonable that a man who made his living as a witch-doctor should say, when asked, that he was a witch-doctor and the man was let off, as I remember, with a small parking fine.

Another thing I'd not anticipated was that as far as the witch-doctors were concerned I had become 'The Man'. I'm not sure how it happened because I've never pretended any great knowledge of witch-doctoring but within months of supplying the first I was supplying many and everything they bought had to be put together by me, personally, because this was an important element in the magic.

As an aside to this it might be worthwhile to offer an alternative view about how the placebo effect works. I guess that the witch-doctors had a subconscious understanding of this process and I often go through it with aromatherapy students and therapists because it seems to me to be an essential understanding for anyone who works in the field of health.

I recently came across a paper which had surprised the medical profession, dealing as it does with placebo surgery. An English surgeon had experimented with a reasonable number of 'knee' patients. One group he performed surgery on. The other group he performed the opening of the skin and the suturing but did no surgery as such. Instead he left them under general anaesthetic for the expected time and played a video of the full procedure as if he was expecting that the sound of the operation, drifting into the subconscious while the body was in this state, might, in itself, have an effect. It did indeed have an effect. The patients who received the placebo surgery fared just as well as the ones who'd actually undergone the operation.

My own view, and this is why I speak to students about this process, is that whether or not the patient believes in the medicine or the procedure is entirely irrelevant. The important factor is that the physician, surgeon or therapist who recommends a particular medicine or course of treatment should expect that the treatment will work. Dr Johnson was the first person to mention this.

The experiment he refers to ran something like this. Johnson was staying the weekend at a country house, the master of which had fallen prey to a mystery illness. He approached the master's manservant who was evidently a few million brain cells short of the full set – which is one of the reasons Johnson singled him out. He gave the servant a curious bottle, which contained only water, but told the man that this was the medicine which would cure his master. He instructed the man to sneak in to his master's bedchamber without waking him and to sprinkle a few drops of the 'magic potion' on the pillow adding that this would effect a cure.

The following morning the master arose hail and hearty, according to Johnson because the servant had 100% certainty that any potion suggested by the great Dr Johnson was sure to work. This experiment fulfilled two criteria. The patient knew nothing about the cure and the person who administered it 'knew' that it was going to work. Recent university research using elegant double-blind trials has confirmed Johnson's suspicion.

In and amongst the witch-doctors, magicians, priests and wizards who frequented the shop were one or two policemen.

On one occasion, a very busy Saturday afternoon, a burly uniformed three-striper with a wonderfully Yorkshire way of delivering police-speak, stepped up to the counter and asked me in a very loud voice "Now then, do you know if it's possible to make wine out of them magic mushrooms?" Fifteen or twenty faces swivelled to look at him and wait for my reply. "I wouldn't like to say, Chief", I said to him, "but as far as I know, it's possible to ferment anything, even old socks. Why don't you try it and let me know how you get on?" There was much smirking around the shop and this one didn't come back.

It was around this time that dittany of Crete became much more easily obtained. Those of us with an interest, because dittany was mentioned in several texts on incense making but had been virtually unobtainable, found ourselves somewhat disappointed when we finally got to set fire to some. It doesn't give off much of an odour at all. However, it does give off massive quantities of dense, grey smoke.

This property came in very handy when a customer asked me to provide something which would provide smoke of such a quality that it could be collected and retained in a plastic bin-liner for a few minutes. It turned out he was a fire training officer and needed to be able to use smoke for a demonstration in a location where naked flame was out of the question. It worked. The trainer came back a few times for more dittany.

A strange old man who may well have been the victim of some hocus pocus himself approached the counter one day and asked if there were any oils which repel flies. I suggested lemongrass and citronella, both of which work reasonably well in different circumstances. After he'd made his choice, it transpired that he had a problem with only one fly which followed him everywhere and even bothered him in his sleep. When I pointed out that there were no flies in the shop he told me in a confidential, almost conspiratorial tone, that it was waiting for him outside.

Only a few days later, I was commissioned to create a scent which probably would have attracted flies quite efficiently, belonging, as it fundamentally did, to the group of odours categorised by perfumers as 'faecal'. My client, on this occasion, was the owner of the waxworks museum in York. He'd recently taken receipt of a yeti and wanted it to smell overpoweringly rancid. I based the creation on artificial civet and asafoetida with a little musk ketone to exalt and bring out the stupefyingly animal nature of the mixture.

The *hocus pocus* element of the shop was not restricted to Christians and witch-doctors. Some of our Muslim clients also had what might be described as 'magical' reasons for using materials they obtained from us. Most curious among these commodities is aloewood which is available both as a wood and as an essential oil.

Aloewood is also known as agar wood, bird wood, eagle wood, el oudh and kaju lakka. The botanical name is *aquilaria agallocha*. I've been unable to ascertain an accurate guesstimate of what the yield of oil from wood might be but it must be infinitesimally small, the annual output of the whole planet amounting to something like five kilos per year. Only mature male trees are felled and it is hoped that much of the heartwood of the tree is fungus infected since it is infection which catalyses the trees production of oil. The wood is chopped into handleable pieces called billets which are thrown into water. Fungus infected wood is denser than non infected wood and sinks. The wood that floats is sent for incense or *agarbatthi* manufacture. The wood that sinks is retained for distillation. This process gave rise to the Chinese name for the oil 'Fragrance sinking under water'.

Aloewood is one of the two aromatic oils which have true animal notes, jasmine being the other. This would make it invaluable in perfumery were it not for the oil's stunning price. On its own it imparts a wonderful, masculine odour which may account for why, in the mythology of Islam, this oil is accounted as being the favourite perfume of the Archangel Michael who is considered to offer, amongst other things, personal protection and guidance. Wearing his favourite perfume attracts Michael to hover around the wearer thereby conferring his benefits.

Aloewood oil is also used in the Middle East to boost the flagging sexual potency of older men (there are many such substances in use for this purpose but none anywhere near so expensive). The oil is heated under a metal plate so that the soot can be collected. This is then consumed. I have heard no reports about the effectiveness of this treatment but I think I would prefer to rely on Michael's ministrations if it were me!

Of all the aromatic commodities available the most extensively used and most widely appreciated in religion/magick/ superstition is frankincense.

To begin with the names:-

Frankincense is derived from the Old French meaning 'real incense'. *Olibanum* (the posh name for this material) is a corruption through the classical languages of the Arabic luban which strictly means 'gum' but, in practice, is always applied to this commodity.

There are actually two forms of frankincense, hard and soft, known in Arabic as *dakr* and *sakr* respectively. *Dakr* is described as male and is used only for incense. *Sakr* is described as female and finds more use in medicines. When I first came across *luban sakr* I thought it so unusual that I bought a kilo of it. With the new find in my hand I visited some friends who owned a perfumery in the bazaar. I wasn't at all prepared for the howls of laughter and the rolling around on the floor which followed my disclosure that the bag contained female frankincense.

When they'd got their breath back and wiped the tears from their eyes, they explained that this type of frankincense is used, almost exclusively by men with erectile problems, and I'd just bought a kilo of it! Like gum mastic, from where comes our word *masticate*, soft frankincense can be chewed. It has no flavour and does not (as chewing gum does) stimulate the production of gastric acids.

Queen Hatshepsut, a Pharaoh of 18th Dynasty Egypt, prized frankincense so highly that she sent an expedition to the land of Punt, present day Somalia, in order to bring back huge quantities of the gum and the living trees. The expedition, led by one San An Mut took three years and is accredited with being proemial to the foundation of the priestly gardens in which medicinal and fragrant plants were studied and used for the next thousand years or more. At Tel El Amarna, the capital of the heretic King Akhnaten, vast quantities of frankincense were burned in the streets to ward off pestilence and to perfume the air.

In present day Egypt, shopkeepers sweeten the pavements outside their premises with the seeds of Syrian rue added to water. Also named *harmal* or *harmine*, this herb achieved fame in the West when it was shown by Alexander Shulgin and others to be a powerful hallucinogen when consumed.

I once bought a kilo of Syrian rue seeds from one of the world-famous herbalists in the Khan El Khalili market in Cairo. It is, indeed a powerful hallucinogen and, while I was experimenting with different preparations of it I discovered that the seed contain a blue oil which is remarkably rare and may indicate the presence of a high proportion of *azulene* which is the active, soothing ingredient in chamomile oils and is probably the element in those oils which kills *staphylococcus aureus*.

The medicinal effects of frankincense were appreciated early in the history of Egypt (as they are to a certain extent today) and it was also used to an extent in the mummification process but its most important function by far was to carry the supplications of the priests to the Gods. This particular use was almost certainly suggested by the contemplative effect of the drug and explains its continued use in churches, mosques and other places of worship.

The Hebrews learned about incense-making from the Egyptians and formulas for their incenses and anointing oils (which rely heavily on frankincense) are to be found in Exodus. The use of the commodities so compounded was strictly forbidden for any use other than intercourse with the God.

Frankincense was at the centre of world trade in pre-classical times and was one of the most precious commodities conceivable. Much of the trade passed through Arabia where high duties were imposed. One theory suggests that this explains the prefix *saudi* which means 'happy'.

The high cost of frankincense is the exoteric reason for its inclusion among the gifts of the Magi. The esoteric explanation is more concerned with priestly ideas of frankincense, its inclusion in the myth of Christ's nativity demonstrating that the child would grow up to be as important as the priest kings of Egypt.

In my early days as a merchant of aromatic commodities, I made the mistake of buying a kilo of frankincense oil from a small company based in London. It was a mistake because the oil smelled like what a colleague of mine who sold good quality frankincense oil described as "a sumo-wrestlers jock-strap".

We live and learn, but it wasn't until years later that I learned that the man who'd sold me the awful stuff worked, during daylight hours, as a chemistry teacher in a London school. In order to keep his buying costs down, he would take a few kilos of frankincense tears into lessons on distillation where each of his students would produce a few grams of oil. This he collected together at the end of the lesson and when he'd accumulated enough, he'd sell the product to naive buyers such as myself.

In later years, having learned my lesson and when business was motoring, I would buy frankincense oil in ten kilo lots, an enormous quantity to buy at one time, considering that such an amount is equivalent to one thousand 10ml bottles.

Traditionally, frankincense is burned on heated metal trays, coal or charcoal but all these methods tend to leave a slightly acrid after-smell because of the impurities in the gum. It is better by far to evaporate the oil (which contains no such impurities), especially during meditation, since it helps to calm and regulate the current of the breath. Production of the oil was first recorded in the drug ordinance of Berlin in 1587.

Sample Incense Formula
1) *Put two ounces of frankincense in a container and add 3ml of oak-moss absolute.*
2) *Mix these substances together.*
3) *If the product is too sticky add a little more frankincense or powdered orris root.*

As I mentioned above, the commodity most often added to frankincense by Christian thurifers is benzoin. The raw material is exuded through the bark of the trunk of the tree, especially where the bark has been incised by the grower. It is this raw material which is used in incense. The oleo-resin, a rectified product which may be liquid at high ambient temperatures is also available.

The name *benzoin* is a perfect example of how the names of some aromatic materials come into being. One might be forgiven for assuming that this commodity has something to do with *benzene* but a little detective work reveals the true origin. In Arabic the name for this resin is *luban jawi* or Javanese gum. The English language has a tendency to compact names so on transfer from one language to the other the initial syllable *lu* was lost. Endings tend to be modified and the j and z sounds in many languages are virtually interchangeable. This reduces *luban jawi* to *banjaw* which is only an etymological step from *benzoin*. *Luban* is applied in Arabic specifically to frankincense whose colour it compares to milk (*laban*).

Benzoin oleo-resin is an extremely viscous material and, especially in cold weather, it can be almost impossible to get out of the bottle. Remove the bottle cap and the dropper if there is one and, with the cap still off, put the bottle somewhere warm – a CH radiator is perfect. You'll probably never be able to coax out one drop but you'll get a small gloop with a bit of practice.

For perfumery purposes, one gram of benzoin added to a litre of ethanol will prepare the alcohol and smooth its edges off in preparation for the addition of essential oils etc. It is also a superb fixative. Because it has a high boiling point it reduces the volatility of any blend to which it is added. Because it has a sweet, balsamic, almost vanilla odour, benzoin oleo-resin finds use in heavy, oriental type perfumes such as chypre. It can also be 'creamed' into powders such as sandalwood to create superb, modern incense.

Somewhat surprisingly, fruits are occasionally used in incenses. Of these, juniperberry, the main flavour component of gin, is perhaps the all time favourite. The essential oil has been used for two hundred years in medicines. However, the history of the plant and berries as a fumigant and incense ingredient stretch back to Ancient Egypt where the berries were one of the ingredients of the notable incense *'Kyphi'* which was burned by the priests of Heliopolis in sacrifice to Kep-Ra, the midnight Sun. A number of formulae for this incense have survived. The following is as good an example as any. The product should be soft and sticky.

Formula for Kyphi Incense
pine resin, wine, galangal root, rush,
juniperberries, broom, mastic, grapes, honey

Kyphi, because of the inclusion of liquids, is better burned on a hot metal plate rather than charcoals. Not exclusively an incense it was also used in poultice form for ulcers etc and may also have been consumed. Certainly while it was still fresh this blend would have been antiseptic and to a certain extent antibiotic.

The use of aromatics in European history, where it is not to do with perfumery, is largely to do with Church, medicine and magic, the three being relatively interchangeable throughout the period between the first crusade and the present. The Church needed consciousness-changing incenses to stupefy its congregations and make them receptive to an inconsistent and repressive dogma. Medicine needed aromatic materials from which to compound poultices, ointments, balsams and so on.

The alchemists/magicians needed aromatics to express the doctrine of signatures (where all things in the cosmos are presumed to vibrate in sympathy, especially with materials and abstracts which belong to their own signature). Thus, if you were that magician, working with a matter of the heart (Venus), you would work in the colour green, using copper tools, smelling of roses. See Aleister Crowley's *777* (tables of correspondences) if you're interested in getting your head into really small spaces.#

The attributed materials and abstracts referred to by The Doctrine of Signatures were never, as it were, standardized. All authorities differ.

Crowley buffs may be interested to know that he bought his animal parts from a Mr Merryweather at Armours in London. His main interest in these items was the making of a perfume called *ruthvah* or the 'perfume of immortality' which contained only the three animal products named above. Immortality was certainly not assured either for the poor animals who lost their lives in the production of this potion (which smelled like sewers to most folk) or for Crowley himself who died at the age of 72.

The attributions listed below for the planets and the signs of the zodiac are as good as any:-

MERCURY	mastic, sandalwood, storax
SATURN	myrrh, civet*
JUPITER	cedar, hyssop
MARS	tobacco, nettle, pepper
SUN	frankincense, acacia, benzoin, bay
VENUS	benzoin, rose, sanderswood
MOON	jasmin, willow, lily
ARIES	dragon's blood, geranium
TAURUS	storax
GEMINI	wormwood, orchid
CANCER	lotus, amber
LEO	frankincense, sunflower
VIRGO	narcissus, lily
LIBRA	galbanum, aloe
SCORPIO	benzoin, opoponax
SAGITTARIUS	lignum aloes, myrrh, civet*
CAPRICORN	musk*, civet*
AQUARIUS	galbanum
PISCES	ambergris*

It must be said that creating zodiac perfumes/incenses from the attributed materials alone is an impossible task in some cases. Even if the materials associated with the ruling planet are brought into use the task remains a difficult one. Those poor guys in The Hermetic Order of the Golden Dawn must have stunk!

Scenting success

RAY SHERWIN'S original bank manager was not keen on the idea at all.

A shop that was going to specialise in selling essential oils for aromatherapy and perfumery did not sound like a very good business venture.

The bank manager reckoned it would not last. "In fact, he promised to expose that which he sits upon at Leeds Town Hall if we were still in business at the end of the first year," said Ray Sherwin.

He and his bank manager parted company and the business, Id Aromatics, has just celebrated its fifth birthday.

Ray, a former English teacher, started experimenting with essential oils and perfume compounds 15 years ago, and the business began as a perfumerie.

Then people began to ask for different oils to use as remedies and there was an increasing interest in aromatherapy, in which essential oils are used.

These aromatic oils are extracted from flowers, leaves, roots and the bark of trees and their beneficial properties have been known for centuries. They can be used as perfumes by themselves, or in bath oils or burned in a fragrancer to perfume the home.

Gently massaged onto the skin they are absorbed into the blood system and can be used for treating skin conditions, boosting the circulation, and easing aches and pains.

Inhaling their vapours can clear the head, nose and chest, and used in the bath they will help you relax. Or if you just want to enjoy the aromas, different oils will have a relaxing or stimulating influence — lemon grass would perk you up and ylang ylang would calm you down.

Many people burn oils for instance while meditating, said Ray, for which he would recommend lavender or frankincense. And others use them for medicinal reasons.

Essential oils are very strong and should not be applied direct to the skin except in miniscule amounts. Massage oils should be made up from a solution consisting of no more than three per cent essential oil to 97 of a carrier or fixing oil such as sweet almond.

Each essence has its own fragrance, properties and peculiarities, explained Ray, and anyone who is interested in using essential oils should understand the individual characteristics of the oils they plan to use.

The Leeds shop, which Ray runs in partnership with Michael Hirst, a former electronics engineer, now stocks more than 200 essential oils.

They still make perfumes and also incenses, the latter for various churches, masonic temples and pagan groups.

So far as they know theirs is the only such shop in any city centre and they attract customers from all over the country as well as abroad.

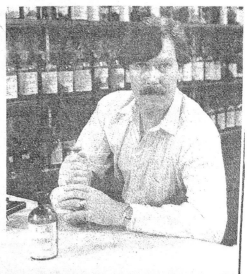

Ray Sherwin in his Leeds shop.

Ray in second Leeds shop, 1986, interviewed by the *Yorkshire Post*, to whom all this was virtually Satan's work at that time.

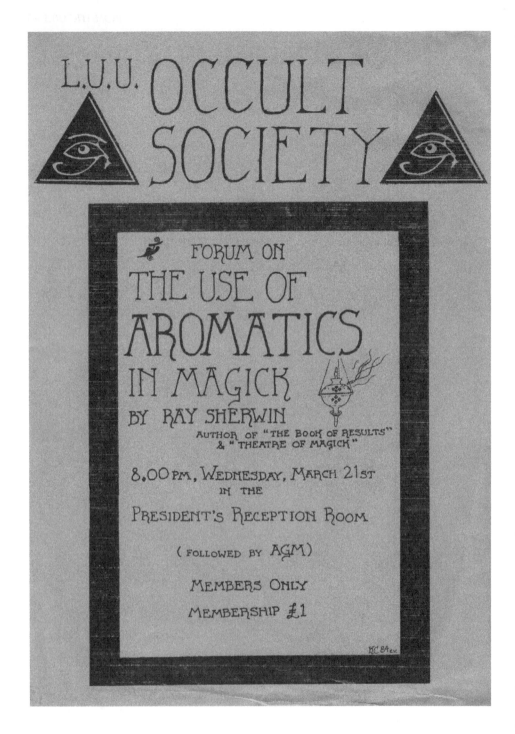

L.U.U. poster for a forum on aromatics. The shop was a favoured meeting place for members who could always rely on a cup of coffee there. Poster designed by Ken Cox who was L.U.U.'s *Grande Fromage* at the time.

Much more promising as a valid exercise in combined perfumery and astrology is the creation of individual fragrances inspired by individual horoscopes. Indeed this would be a welcome shift away from the product-oriented tightness of control required by both the Doctrine of Signatures and the fragrance industry. The Doctrine really would like to be able to put everything in the cosmos into a 'correct' pigeon-hole. The fragrance industry would like us all to smell like product. Individuality of smell is something we all possess by birthright although many of us don't have the olfactory refinement to distinguish between individuals. What we embellish our personal smell with is up to us – we have the essential oils.

It would be remiss to end the *hocus pocus* tale without mentioning that Leeds, during the 1980s, enjoyed an 'occult revival' reminiscent of the occult explosion which took place in London over the turn of the nineteenth and twentieth centuries. In London at that time the big league players were The Theosophical Society, The Hermetic Order of the Golden Dawn and the various organisations associated with Aleister Crowley.

In 1980s Leeds the main player was the newly emerging Chaos Magick which, despite its somewhat barbarous sounding name sought to bring pragmatism and thorough research into the realms of self-study and development. Indeed, it was an exciting time with massive interest being focussed on Chaos Magick groups and on the University Occult Society. My own little claim to fame is to be found in one of the magazines from this period which sought, in a spoof article, to find definitions appropriate to the surnames of some of the folk who were prominent on the Leeds occult scene at that time. Accordingly, a Sherwin was defined as '**the strange smell in the car**' on the way home from a ritual.

It was also at about that time that a book I'd written several years earlier started to become quite popular. *The Book of Results* sought to clarify and develop a technique which had been pioneered a few decades earlier by an artist and sorcerer named Austin Osman Spare. The technique, known as sigilisation, is a way of making spells and designing them to fit particular purposes.

I'd been introduced to the theories of Austin Osman Spare by Pete Carroll, a writer who contributed frequently to *The New Equinox*, a magazine I edited and published in the 1970s. The purpose of *The New Equinox* was to make available, on the cheap, treatises on occultism which had become very rare or prohibitively expensive. I duly included some of the works of Austin Spare and became interested in his work almost immediately.

One of the ways in which I developed Spare's technique was to suggest that the sense of smell had been unreasonably overlooked by just about everyone who'd written on the subject of self-metaprogramming. In fact, as other sections of this book point out, smell impacts on the subconscious in amazing ways which are, actually, not difficult to understand.

What strikes me as peculiar now, more than thirty years after the first publication of *The Book of Results* is that the book is still selling. Would that my music and poetry were so popular.

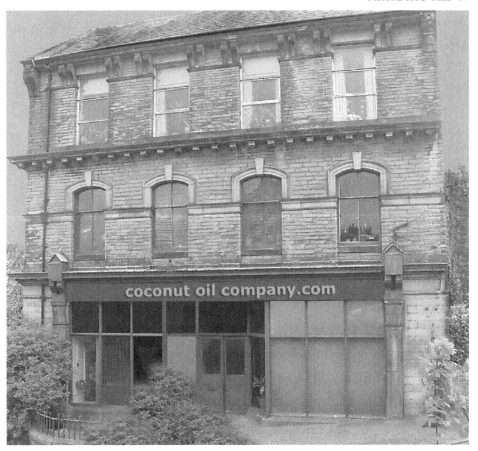

The Hermitage, 2009. Now specialising in importing and distributing virgin coconut oil, I'm still enthusiastic about essential oils and do some product development and a little supply.

When Aleister Crowley came across a literary reference to an excellent curry he'd once made, he wrote on the fly leaf

'On Crowley the immortals ironically look,
He sought fame as a poet, and found it as a cook.'
(I know the feeling.)

In recent books there has been a great deal of speculation about where Chaos Magick came about. Some say there was a secret enclave in Whitby, others that the founders of the movement met in a shop in Leeds.

In fact, Pete Carroll and I first met in Deptford where he occupied a squat in Speedwell House. Later Pete moved to East Morton, about a hundred metres from my place. This gave us lots of opportunity to plot and experiment with ether and other mind alterants, favourite amongst which was probably beer. We also had a lot of fun with explosives such as hydrogen and ammonium tri-iodide. A few years later, Pete went on to open an aromatics shop in Bristol.

Ambergris is a pathological secretion of the sperm-whale and was extensively used in former times as a fixative and toner for perfumes. While whaling is still carried out by Norwegian and Japanese barbarians it is very important for us not to use it. When whaling is a thing of the past, all ambergris appearing on the market will be 'found' and consequently usable.

Please use synthetics of the animal substances. The natural commodities are responsible for a great deal of senseless suffering amongst sperm-whales (ambergris), civet cats (civet)

and musk deer (musk). In addition, they are expensive, difficult to obtain and tiresome to process into anything like a useable state. Nature-identical synthetics are available and are ready-to-use.

3

Ritual Magick for the BBC

In 1987 I was visited by a television producer who worked for the BBC. He had a problem. At that time BBC2 was running a series of community based programmes which were largely self-made by groups who had some sort of an axe to grind.

The producer, whose name was Paul, had been approached by a vicar of the shake-your-tambourine-for-Jesus type, who wanted to make a programme about the horrifying number of covens and satanic groups whose adherents were beginning to outnumber the God-fearing folk of Lancashire.

Actually, Paul had two problems. The first was that, although the makers of all the other programmes in the series had been allowed to make their films as they wished, he obviously couldn't let the loony vicar say anything he liked so, for this programme only, he wanted to present the film maker's point of view alongside a reasoned but opposite point of view. Otherwise the whole series would have come into disrepute.

The second problem was that, with the exception of a few eccentrics and a handful of intelligent men who'd been filmed in derelict places talking sensibly about life, the universe and everything, Paul hadn't been able to find anyone to film or interview.

In desperation, he came to see me - in darkest Yorkshire. He needed some footage of 'Pagan' activity to counterbalance scenes filmed in the church at the centre of the programme. At that time I was working with a dedicated group of people who were all interested in using the glamour or theatre of ritual Magick to explore possibilities and potentials. Our problem, as far as Paul's dilemma was concerned, was that we all wanted to remain anonymous and we didn't want our premises to appear on television.

We were also well aware that if we offered lots of footage, the producer and editor would be able to make of it whatever they pleased. After a lot of thought I came up with a solution that suited everyone.

I told Paul that we weren't prepared to be filmed in our usual place of working and that we weren't prepared to be filmed performing an actual ritual. What we would do was dress up theatrically and present him with some Denis Wheatley style footage. Altogether we would give him about three minutes' worth of material. This met with Paul's enthusiastic approval. In fact, we'd decided that the opportunity to perform an experiment with six million people potentially taking part, was too good an opportunity to miss.

The appointed night was excruciatingly cold and we'd agreed that a rocky outcrop near the top of Ilkley Moor would be a nicely atmospheric location. The last mile or so had to be walked. For us that meant carrying our costumes and props. For the crew it meant lugging cameras, tripods and the lighting rig.

By the time we were half-way there, I realised that there was ice forming in my ears. My moustache and eyebrows had whitened giving a bizarre 'Scott of the Antarctic' impression. One of my colleagues, who had very long hair at the time pointed out that it was frozen solid.

When the lighting and sound checks had been done we presented our three minutes of 'pretend' ritual. What we presented him with, in fact, was a group sigilisation, a kind of spell, whose aim was to end the threat of nuclear war. Why not aim for something big in this circumstance? In the final seconds, a banner with a design which unmistakably expressed our purpose, was burned. The intention of the ritual was, undoubtedly, shared subconsciously by many of the viewing audience.

Then we packed up and drank the two bottles of vodka which the BBC expenses had provided. By that time we were all desperate for anti-freeze, but very pleased that the many rehearsals we'd done had paid off with a slick performance and split-second timing.

The programme was aired on BBC2 in 1987 under the title 'Lucifer over Lancashire'.

4

A Spooky Aside

By the time Michael and I had been running the shop for eight years or so, we both started to feel the need for a change. Michael's intention was to use his part of his share of the money raised by selling the business to buy and convert a fifty-three seater coach into a mobile home in which he and his wife, Jill, would live permanently. That was in 1990 and they are still, at the time of writing (2009) living in the same bus!

My intention was to continue working with essential oils but to drop all the peripheral stuff such as candles, incense, evaporators and so on. In other words, I'd determined to specialize.

A few years earlier I'd bought a large building in the village which had been built by The Co-operative Society in the 1860s. Originally my idea was to convert it and live in it. By the time I'd done that I still had two floors left over so, most conveniently, I had a place from which to operate my new business *Hermitage Oils*, without even having to leave the house.

I'd already been living in Morton for ten years when I bought the building which I mischievously re-named *The Hermitage*. Until that time I'd always referred to the building in the same way as the other locals. They called it "'T' aunted Quorp", or, in comprehensible English "The haunted Co-op". The place had been much more than a shop that had occupied only the ground floor. Above it was warehousing and an office. Above that was the original Village Institute, complete with a stage, a boxing ring, a vaulting-horse and a readers' corner. But it was the original use of the basement which originally gave rise to the building's spooky nickname.

From the time when the building was erected and for a hundred years the basement had been the village mortuary. There were still stone laying-out tables in there when I moved in, twenty-five years after The Co-op had departed. When the mortuary had been in use there had been a macabre notification system which must have enhanced the reputation of the place enormously. The way it worked was this. If one of your family died during the night, you would go to The Co-op and write the name and address of the deceased on a coffin-shaped blackboard which stood outside. Not only did this alert the morticians, it informed the rest of the village too!

Considering that I live and work above an old mortuary and

undertakery, I must admit that I've never experienced anything at all out of the ordinary. Except once. Here's the tale.

I bought the building from an electrical engineering company who'd occupied it for twenty-five years. While contracts were being sorted out ready for completion to take place, I asked the boss if he'd ever encountered any non-corporeal residents. The only thing he'd been impressed by didn't make a very good story in itself. He'd been working late one night on a circuit board when the telephone rang. He had a brief conversation with the caller and then hung-up the receiver and turned back to his work. The blue-handled side-cutters he'd been using had disappeared. He looked everywhere but couldn't find the tool he'd put down a few moments earlier. He'd not moved from his seat but the cutters were nowhere to be found.

Some years later, after Michael and Jill had departed on their bus, I was converting the ground floor into offices and work rooms ready to begin trading as *Hermitage Oils*. One corner of the office was boxed in and I thought this area would be a good site for a work-station. If the panelling were removed there'd be space for a console, a printer and so on, so I set to with a crowbar, removing the panelling which The Co-op people had but there one hundred and twenty-five years earlier. When I pulled off the last panel, there, on one of the cross-members was a pair of blue-handled side-cutters. I could feel the small hairs on my neck begin to stand up! The side-cutters are still in my tool box and I'm working right now at the work-station that was created when the panelling was removed.

5

A Rose by Any Other Name...

The sense of smell and the human animal

One of the most difficult things to come to terms with within the disciplines of aromatherapy and perfumery is the extreme concentration of the raw materials used. The power of essential oils is thrown into sharp relief when compared with the smells that we human beings produce ourselves and the effects that these smells bring about in others even at threshold or 'unsmellable' concentrations.

In evolutionary terms the sense of smell was already fully developed by the time that man arrived on the scene. Had it not been so man might not have survived since it was his sense of smell more than any other which was responsible for choosing safe foods, identifying enemies and for controlling mating and birthing. It was only from the relatively recent time of man's becoming conscious of himself, when the senses of sight and hearing began to come into predominance, that the sense of smell became less important in terms of survival of the species and consequently less refined and less acute.

For modern man the sense of smell hardly functions as a survival mechanism at all except, for example, as an early warning of fire or gas escape, or to detect 'off-notes' in food which has been badly stored or ill-prepared. Until the 1960s people might have been forgiven for believing that the nose was simply an organ of pleasure whose only functions were to sniff up voluptuous odours and to act as an adjunct to the taste buds, but research carried out over the last thirty years is beginning to re-establish the sense of smell as being at least equal in importance to the other senses.

With the possible exception of touch our other senses are trained into sophistication by our parents, our schooling and through the activities we choose to carry out. Few people enjoy wine or strong cheese until they have 'acquired' the taste for them and this applies to many of the substances we enjoy eating and drinking. Perspective is a skill which has to be learned and there are many people outside of western culture who never learn it because their world contains no straight lines. As very young infants we learn to distinguish the phonemes and morphemes which constitute language. Abilities such as this are acquired gradually over a number of years. We tend to refine our senses of touch only when we need to as in the case of someone gone blind who then needs the sensitivity of touch required to read Braille.

The sense of smell, by and large, is developed only by people who need to use it in their work. Wine-blenders and perfumers are cases par excellence but although their skill is appreciated by the people who use their products that appreciation is limited by an uneducated sense of smell. In this case beauty really is in the nostril of the sniffer!

In terms of our relationships with each other it is the effect of smells at a subliminal level which is most interesting. Smells too weak to be noticed by even the most educated nose have their effect on the brain behind that nose without the slightest conscious recognition that the individual is responding to a biological stimulus.

As an example of this:- The stress levels of test subjects were measurably raised when a concentration of 'the smell of hospitals' too weak to be consciously acknowledged by the nose was sprayed into their comfortable environment.

It is a bizarre fact of nature that sows root for truffles because that fungus chemically mimics the smell of the boar. When the sow digs it out the truffle's spores are distributed to places they would not otherwise have reached. Further with respect to pigs, it was discovered in the early seventies that the boar produces a pheromone (external chemical messenger) which acts as a mating stimulant to the sow through the sense of smell and which, although the odour is hardly perceptible, recalls the scent of truffles. This pheromone can be artificially produced and has been used with success by pig breeders to prepare reluctant sows for mating.

Of more immediate interest to the general reader is that

because pigs are biologically similar to humans the pheromone used by pig breeders has a similar effect on people. A man who wears that pheromone like a perfume will attract women to him despite the fact that his 'perfume' is all but undetectable to most of the people in his environment. An unfortunate side-effect is that the same substance tends to make other men aggressive towards the wearer. The human male no longer needs to resort to 'Boarmate' since *androstenone*, the human male equivalent, is now contained, somewhat unwisely in my opinion, in a number of proprietary after-shaves.

At the time that the research into porcine pheromones was getting into full swing it was revealed by another team of researchers that a certain type of moth was able to detect a potential mate eight miles up wind entirely through the action of pheromones and, rather more sinister, *New Scientist* magazine reported that a researcher who had been making headway into the synthesis of artificial musks (fragrance enhancers) had been closed down by the government, his research confiscated.

Exciting though all that was, a lot seems to have happened since those days. It is now suspected that there are at least two hundred distinguishable compounds in human body odours. When Walt Whitman wrote the immortal line 'The scent of these armpits, aroma finer than prayer' he can hardly have been aware that he was praising the aromatic virtues of pheromones blended with fatty acids boofed up by the action of bacteria. A few of these odourous cocktails are worthy of individual mention.

Trimethylamine is produced by the action of bacteria on the nitrogen in the nooks and crannies of the skin. At its strongest it receives descriptions comparing it to rank seafood and according to one source it may be among the most primitive smells we know. It is certainly one of the predominant smells of menstruation among the racial groups who consume copious fatty acids as part of their diet - meat, dairy products etc. Some people, both male and female, cannot smell TMA at all. Others can detect the smell at one two-thousandth of the concentration required by others and this, of course, has dramatic effects on personal relationships.

A man who picks up TMA at below the threshold level and who has an adverse reaction to it is not likely to get on at an intimate level with a woman whose TMA output is high. Flavourings manufactured through the action of salt and fermentation on sea foods such as oysters and prawns contain TMA (one reason for the reputation of sea-foods as aphrodisiacs?), minute amounts of which, added to cooked dishes impart a savouriness in the same way that asafoetida, which is absolutely disgusting by itself, substantially improves the flavour of curry when used below the threshold level.

Iso-valeric acid, in the sweat of the palms and soles, is another component of essential oil of humans. It is repulsive in concentration but at the threshold level may be one of the important chemical stimuli for mating to occur since its production by the human female rises to a peak at mid-cycle when she is at her most fertile. The presence of IVA in a number of renowned cheeses may explain their popularity.

Esters of *para amino benzoic acid* are found mostly between the toes and, presumably by coincidence, mimic the vaginal smells of a bitch in season. My feet are always clean and, to all intents, odour free but a friend of mine once had a dog that was content to lick between my toes for hours on end without any evident signs of disappointment. Could this be one of the reasons for the long history of co-operation and amity between dog and man?

Exclusive to men is *pyrroline* which gives semen its characteristic odour and which is also distributed by the pubic hair. Although it goes undetected by one in six individuals its contribution to the overall 'human essence' is undeniable. There are, for example, many components of perfumes which are undetectable in the finished product which, none the less, would leave the perfume much poorer in their absence.

Exclusive to women is *dodecanol*, a soapy, fruity odorant dispersed by the breath of ovulating women and there are the so-called 'copulins', controlled by oestrogen, which smell fatty or sweaty but which are not unpleasant at the threshold level. Of rather different function is *isobutyraldehyde*, a milky, somewhat malty smell which guides the new born child to mother's nipple.

Plants produce essential oils largely for two reasons. To attract the right kind of insect for pollination and to discourage insect and animal enemies. The human essences are produced for the same reasons - to attract a mate and, in the case of *androstenone* (actually a group of similar chemicals) to warn off potential competition. Given that these chemical signals are almost exclusively sexual it is not surprising that the production of some of them is increased during sexual arousal or coitus and that the appreciation of the fragrances so created is quite different from other times. TMA might not smell so good especially if it is very strong but during the act of love it is more than acceptable, it is positively aphrodisiac.

In the absence of *testosterone* which controls male and, to a lesser extent, female pheromone production, the sense of smell may not be present at all as though nature has decided that if the individual is unable to reproduce there's no reason for him to have a good sense of smell either. In fact, the inability to smell is often accompanied by loss of sexual appetite in both men and women and sometimes by impotence.

Modern living inhibits the action of pheromones. We wear clothes which contain them rather than allowing them to radiate from our bodies as would naturally be the case. Assisting this process of radiation is the body hair.

When a hair stands up on end it can be literally pumping body essences into the air but the tendency of English and American women to depilate their bodies abandons this function. Indeed, it may be that depilation is carried out, not to enhance the appearance of the body as is invariably the stated reason but to reduce the likelihood of sexual advances by limiting pheromone output.

Strong synthetic perfumes have been fashionable for the past sixty years or so. The public has presumed that these are attractive to the opposite sex but it may well be that they 'drown out' the natural attractants produced by the body.

The healthy, clean human body produces, along with pheromones, its own natural perfumes. There is no reason why these should not be supplemented with delicate natural perfumes but there is nothing so offensive as being able to smell someone's perfume from six feet away. This kind of audacity is like playing one's hi-fi so loud that the neighbours can't hear their canary sing.

We get smell-bombarded in other ways too. Many household products such as washing powder, boot polish, soap and shampoo are so unsubtly perfumed that they represent assault and battery of the olfactory system. Since the way our environment smells can strongly affect the way we feel we need to pay just as much attention to it as we do to the way we smell ourselves.

A true hedonist, I rejoiced at the introduction of bio-degradable washing-up liquids not just because they were eco-friendly but also because the delicate essential oils used by the manufacturers to perfume them made me glad to do the dishes.

There are, of course, other ways in which smells have their effect on us. The odours of childhood and the languorous scents of distant countries bring moods and memories flooding back even when we don't consciously recognise what's going on.

In considering the ways in which human behaviour is modified by smells in the environment there are two, reasonably distinct approaches. For my own convenience I label these 'personal' and 'biological'.

The 'personal' is concerned with the ways in which incidents from the individual's past become tied up in memory with the smells that were in the environment at the time of the incident. Simple examples of this:- lilacs remind those of us from temperate climes of springtime; cow-shit reminds us of the countryside. These are personal reminiscences being stimulated by current time smells.

The picture becomes more convoluted when the incidents and smells are truly personal. Example:- a boy's first romantic encounter is in a hay barn (OK, it's a bit D H Lawrence but it provides a good illustration). The man's libido is thereafter stimulated by the smells of hay, slightly decaying vegetable matter and rusty agricultural equipment as well as the subtle pheromones and similar compounds discussed previously.

This is not an intellectual thing. The feelings arise without any conscious awareness of the process taking place, rather like subliminal advertising. This mechanism appears to work on many different levels, the unpleasant as well as the pleasant. In Freudian terms a *complex* has been created. Whether you agree with the Freudian model or not this comparison helps us to understand how a tangle of smells, experienced at different times in the past, can exert an effect on emotions and behaviour in the present.

The director of a version of Gorky's play *Summer Folk*, which ran at The Bradford Playhouse for a couple of weeks, understood this principle well enough to invite me to perfume the auditorium with the scents of flowers appropriate to the different parts of spring and summer in which the protagonists have picnics together. At that time there were no electronic evaporators - we didn't do that until 1988.

The brass and stoneware evaporators we were having manufactured for us ran on candle power, and health and safety regulations forbade their use in a theatre. I hit on a simple expedient. At given cues I would put a few drops of the appropriate flower oil on a tissue and put this between the central heating radiator grills throughout the auditorium. Within seconds, the perfume filled the place and, along with clever lighting and scenery, enhanced 'the effect of being there'.

Of course, there are human odours I've not mentioned. I make reference to farting here only because my friends would be confounded if I didn't.

A close friend of mine emigrated to Australia and, while he was finding his feet there, he took on any job that came his way. One of these jobs was working as a waiter for the Freemasons.

There were, my friend delighted in telling me, occasional ultra-posh dinners which took place in the enormous round, with the waiters toffed up in red tail-coats and bow ties. Between serving courses, the many waiters stood in the 'at ease' position with the hands clasped behind the back.

'The technique' had been faithfully passed on to each newly recruited waiter. It was simple, but devastating. Each waiter would practice continence in the gas department until the main speech started. Then, hands already appropriately positioned, he would surreptitiously part his buttocks to ensure that no tell-tale sounds accompanied the emission. With fifteen or more enthusiasts making a concerted effort, and with no obvious source for the rapid and unpleasant rise in atmospheric levels of sulphurous toxins and skatol, the speaker was evidently often perplexed as to why his audience was suddenly grimacing or, on especially successful occasions, leaving.

6

The Fats of Life

What your mother would have told you if she'd known

In the early eighties while I was running the shop, evening primrose oil was beginning to attract attention because of its gamma linolenic (omega 3) acid content. I duly studied it and started to sell it. Despite having no background in chemistry it was evident to me that EPO by itself would oxidise as soon as it was swallowed so I added an anti-oxidant.

The thought never crossed my mind, and indeed it is a thought which seems to have evaded everyone else's minds too, that all unsaturated oils need to have an anti-oxidant added to them, otherwise they become, or in some cases ARE, rancid.

More than twenty years later when I found out that my thyroid had virtually packed up, naturally I wanted to research the subject so that I could understand the problem and make whatever modifications to my lifestyle that might be called for. The information that I came up with, largely concerning oil (dietary fat) was disconcerting in several ways.

As a vegan I'm obviously concerned about what I eat and as someone who's worked in the field of holistic health for more than twenty years I'm of the opinion that you are what you eat. My recent researches have demonstrated to me that this old adage is true and, lately, in some very scary ways (of which more later).

I can't remember (a thyroid problem!) who it was who made the following brilliant observation but I often use it as a start point when I'm getting to grips with a health problem, mine or someone else's.

The proposition is this: If your body is not working properly it's because:

1. **You're putting something into it that should not be there.**
2. **You're not putting something into it that should be there.**
3. **There is something in your environment which is causing you a problem (and I would include genetic factors here).**

My first task, then, was to find out if there were any foods which are antagonistic to the function of the thyroid. There are and, I must admit, I was not at all pleased with the information I turned up. The number one thyroid antagonist is peanuts and peanut butter both of which belonged, until recently, in the category of 'my favourite foods'.

No problem – there are many other nuts some of which are much more nutritionally important – walnuts are a rich source of omega 3s, brazils are a rare provider of selenium. In fact peanuts are legumes, much more closely related to peas than to nuts.

What I found next was much more disconcerting, especially for a vegan, until I came upon the solution. There is a group of foods which is antagonistic toward thyroid function and this group has come to be known as *vegetable oils*. The group includes, as main culprits, seed oils such as sunflower, safflower, canola (rape seed) with soya oil strongly suspected.

These oils and peanuts and peanut oil are referred to as goitregens because of their antagonism towards thyroid function. When I commented to my doctor that I'd removed all the goitregens from my diet his less than encouraging response was "What are goitregens?" As an aside, I must comment, for the benefit of anyone who is interested in hypothyroidism, that iodine, while it is essential for thyroxine (thyroid hormone) production, is a goitregen itself if too much is consumed.

OK. So that's me sorted out in terms of what I should not eat but am I really going to have to start eating animal fats? I've not had anything to do with them for years, not only for ethical reasons but also because of the raft of toxins and dodgy proteins associated with them. Despite recent fad diets aimed at virtually fat-free eating, most authorities on nutrition reckon that between 20% and 30% of caloric intake should be as fat. So, are there any other alternatives?

Fortunately there are. Virgin olive oil is reasonably stable if it's not taken up to cooking temperatures but actually finding a source of truly cold pressed, untreated olive oil is very difficult. My research turned up two fats which are stable at cooking temperatures. The first of these, palm oil, I ruled out for my own use because of the huge tracts of forest being destroyed in order to create plantations; a good nutrient, unavailable to me for reasons other than nutrition. This leaves one fat and, fortunately, it's the best of the lot. Coconut oil.

Before I go on, it would be expedient to define the difference between oil and fat since this is a potential confusion. The difference is simple. A vegetable fat is nothing more than an oil which is solid at room temperature. As far as coconut is concerned, because it melts at 76 degrees Fahrenheit, it is an oil in some parts of the world and a fat in others. Coconut butter is a reference to the oil in its semi-solid state.

Coconut oil has been virtually ignored as a nutrient because it is a saturated fat. In the 1950s an American researcher, Ancel Keyes, came up with what was to be called 'The Lipid Hypothesis'. It was this hypothesis which instigated the whole 'low-fat' craze. The suggestion was straight forward enough. Saturated fat, it claimed, leads to high levels of cholesterol and high cholesterol levels lead to cardio-vascular disease.

It did not take account of other factors such as low vitamin C status (an idea championed by Nobel laureate Linus Pauling). Nor did it take account of the fact that there are, basically, three types of saturated fat, short, medium and long chain, with the medium chain group, which includes coconut and palm oils, having many wonderful nutrient and medicinal properties.

(As far as I can make out, cholesterol is part of the cardio-vascular system's self-repair mechanism and the notion of forcing down abnormally high levels of it is analogous to removing the belts and air-bags from your car because they remind you that accidents are possible or taking the police off the streets in high crime areas).

It appears to have been the media more than the medics or nutritionists who pushed the Lipid Hypothesis at the public, no doubt encouraged by the producers of seed oils (unsaturates and polyunsaturates) who, until that time had only been able to sell their products into the paints and varnishes industry.

In fact, at just about that time, manufacturers of paints and varnishes were beginning to look to petroleum derivatives as drying agents in their products and the seed oil producers were facing what must have seemed to them like a total commercial void since there were no other major applications for their product other than the manufacture of traditional linoleum (linseed aka flax seed oil) and oil painting (linseed and other unsaturates are all 'drying' oils).

The Lipid Hypothesis remains just that. A shot in the dark. It has never been proved. On the contrary, demographic studies (examinations of populations) have shown that there seems to be no connection at all between saturated fats and disease. At the turn of the nineteenth into the twentieth century, for example, saturated fat constituted 95% of the total fat intake of people in the western world, yet heart disease *and cancer* were extremely rare.

The famous Seven Countries study found that the people of Japan and Crete were longest lived despite their intake of saturated fat being higher than any of the other people surveyed. It is now strongly suspected that Ancel Keyes chose his own countries to demonstrate the Lipid Hypothesis but despite the fact that this puts his work into total disrepute, his hypothesis is still the basis of the chorus to avoid saturated fat.

Unsaturates and polyunsaturates are distinguished by having one pair or more of double carbon bonds. These bonds are, as it were, incomplete and readily attach oxygen or hydrogen molecules to themselves. That is, they readily oxidise or hydrogenate. Oxidative stress on the body is a major cause of disease. This *may* be why these oils have such a negative effect on the thyroid, contributing greatly to the current explosion of obesity as a disease in itself. In my view it is *certainly* one of the major causes of cancer and this is why we are constantly being reminded about foods and supplements which have an anti-oxidant value.

The best word to describe unsaturates and polyunsaturates is 'rancid'. They are rancid by nature, more rancid if they are stored and more rancid yet if they are taken up to cooking temperatures. A perfectly fresh oil from this category will oxidise as soon as it is swallowed. There is worse to come. Food manufacturers, seeking alternatives to the now demonised lard and butter came up with hydrogenated vegetable oils. These are the same oils but have had hydrogen passed through them to stabilise the carbon bonds by attaching a hydrogen molecule. This has the effect of packing the structure of the oil more closely together, thereby creating shortening – a substance which is solid at room temperature.

Here comes the scary part. The body needs saturated fat for cell-wall integrity. However, it seems that the body cannot distinguish between saturated fats and hydrogenated oils (pseudo-saturated fats)/unsaturates. Either that or, in the absence of saturated fat, the body has to make the most of what it can get. This means that cell-wall integrity in individuals who eat hydrogenated oils and unsaturates is compromised. Pigs and rats, better informed by their nervous systems than humans, but scavengers *par excellence*, will have nothing to do with hydrogenated oils. Furthermore, recent research indicates that hydrogenated oils play a part in the incidence of Alzheimer's and other very serious diseases.

Keeping this in mind it is difficult to make sense of the official advice to mothers given in the USA regarding infant formula milk. Despite the fact that mother's milk is 50% fat and very high in cholesterol, which is what the child needs for proper development, particularly of the brain, American 'specialists', advise the use of low-fat, low-cholesterol formula. There is, incidentally, a chemical similarity between the fat in mother's milk and the fat found in coconut oil. They are both medium chain fatty acids rich in lauric acid and help the body ward off viral, bacterial and fungal infections of various types. The body converts lauric acid into monolaurin, a substance which has even greater anti-microbial effectiveness.

My interest in coconut oil as a nutrient was fired up when I came across a strange fragment in the history of pig husbandry. In the 1950s, American pig farmers, forever on the lookout for cheap ways to fatten up their livestock began adding coconut oil to the pigs normal feed. A low cost, saturated fat, they presumed, would fatten their animals in double quick time without costing a great deal. Unfortunately the venture did not work out. The more coconut oil the pigs were fed, the leaner they got and the trials were abandoned. The farmers then turned to polyunsaturates and watched the piggy pounds pile on. Not only are these oils intrinsically more fattening than coconut (9 kcal per gm as opposed to 8.3 kcal per gm), because they are thyroid antagonists they slow down the metabolisation of all the food eaten.

Subsequent studies found that pigs fed on small quantities of polyunsaturates were fat by the end of their lives in comparison with pigs fed on large quantities of coconut oil which remained lean and active until the end. In fact, by 1950 it had been demonstrated that unsaturates interfere with thyroid function by blocking the function of thyroid transport protein as well as by interfering with the action of digestive enzymes in the stomach. Thyroxine is formed in the thyroid gland by the action of the same enzyme. Unsaturates inhibit that enzyme and the more unsaturated an oil is the greater the damage it causes.

In a bizarre twist of fortune which has not been generally reported, lard rendered from pigs or other animals which have been fed vegetable oils cannot be recognised as saturated! Since the human body requires high amounts of saturated fat, even the meat which most people are eating is not fulfilling this basic requirement.

Coconut oil doesn't only help to keep one slim because its caloric value is lower than other fats. Because it is a medium chain fatty acid it is taken up by the blood stream and transported directly to the liver where it is converted into energy much as carbohydrate is. What this means is that, so long as you're not eating too much to cover your energy requirements you can add coconut to the equivalent of 250kcal per day and still lose weight! Wow! It also stimulates the thyroid. When I first started using it for cooking and spreading I went red for two days as my metabolic rate was stepped up.

The British government periodically announces that it's about to spend a great deal more money on the National Health Service. It announces this because more money for the Health Service is a vote winner. I despair when I hear these announcements at the further waste of money. That may not sound like a caring person's attitude. Let me explain what I mean.

Government seeks to show how successfully it is coping with increasing health problems by telling us how many more people were treated this year. Now if I were benign dictator of Great Britain I would measure the success of the Health Service by how many fewer people needed to be treated than in the previous year.

We know many of the reasons for the epidemic of cancers. Spending huge amounts of money to find a magic bullet to cure them is little more than a sop to the markets. They create the cancers with their pollution and Frankenstein foods and then want us to pay again for 'research'.

"Prevention is better than cure" sounds like a platitude because we hear it so often. But if we got the phthalates and other oestrogen-like compounds out of our water supply, if we got the PCBs and methyl mercury out of the fish (and fish oils!) and if the Food Standards Agency did a proper job by defining what food is and then forbidding the rest (hydrogenated oils, polyunsaturates etc) WE WOULD NOT NEED TO DO CANCER RESEARCH.

The way that governments support the tobacco industry is a blatant example of the way in which they protect the economic interests of their supporters as priority, disregarding common sense and basic humanity. Adolf Hitler, about whom I have only one good thing to say (and this is it) established an institute in 1930s Germany to find out why so many of the Master Race were dying from lung-cancer. Within a couple of years the report came back to him that tobacco smoking was just about the only cause. Because Hitler's primary concern in this matter was The Race rather than economics he immediately embarked on a 'No Smoking' campaign which was so successful that by the end of the war the Germans smoked less than any other country in the developed world.

When the Americans overran Germany they discovered the research findings of Hitler's cancer research institute but, because Americans are primarily concerned with economics, they managed to keep the findings secret until 1964 by which time the cat was out of the bag anyway.

When Berlin was partitioned by the Russians and the beleaguered West Berliners were critically short of food, medicines and other basic supplies the merciful Berlin Airlift began. Of all the necessities required in West Berlin the Americans ensured that the first cargo to arrive was eighty tons of tobacco. John F Kennedy's famous statement of twenty years later "Ich bin ein Berliner" sounds rather hollow in the light of that information.

The Americans were interested, first and foremost in re-establishing a market-place for tobacco which had been flagging because of Herr Hitler's pesky interference. It is strange to consider that the American and British tobacco pushers have killed many more people than Adolf Hitler did, yet we permit them to continue plying their horrendous trade and even afford the barons of the 'industry' respect. My respect will go to the first supermarket chain to declare the sale of tobacco products unethical.

In Britain the diseases such as lung cancer which are directly connected with smoking tend to affect people in later life. From the government's point of view, especially since the government makes more money out of tobacco than the 'industry' itself, this is brilliant. Get the people onto tobacco, make £3.00 tax on every packet of twenty while the person is healthy and working. Come retirement age the smoker is just about ready to shuffle off the mortal coil thereby neatly sidestepping the need for the state to pay a pension.

When I started writing this the British Prime Minister occupied the bottom of a deep hole with respect to his decision to support the American junta in its illegal invasion of Iraq. Eighteen months later, unable to justify the invasion for the given reasons for going in, he was forced to play the joker of 'human rights'. By 'coalition' reckoning Sadam Hussein killed 30,000 of his own people, principally using poison gas supplied by the Americans, although this last point is seldom reported.

Tobacco kills 126, 000 people per year in Great Britain alone, but the Prime Minister even backtracked on his pre-government promise to ban tobacco advertising on the Grand Prix circuit (in order to protect a regular, large donation to the New Labour Party). In fact, it was revealed in 2008 that Harold MacMillan, Prime Minister in the fifties, deliberately concealed the mounting evidence that cigarette use was directly linked to lung-cancer, fearing that tax revenues would be adversely affected.

If an alien were to look at the tobacco situation he would find it very perplexing. Unqualified people at virtually every street corner selling an extremely dangerous drug to people who then inflict it on others by smoking virtually anywhere they please while other, much more benign drugs are either illegal or available only on prescription.

If we, as people rather than as the components of a marketplace, were truly concerned about cancer we would take tobacco products out of the corner shops, garages and supermarkets so that our children were not exposed to them at all. The same remarks apply to alcohol.

My proposition is this; that all drugs of 'leisure'* – tobacco, alcohol, heroine, LSD, MDMA (aka ecstacy), opium, amphetamine etc., should be sold through a chain of specialist government shops. I have deliberately omitted cannabis from this list because it contains no alkaloid (eg morphine, cocaine, heroine, caffeine and other 'ines') and cannot realistically be considered to be a drug at all. It is more sensibly considered to be a herb.

---

*It is interesting to note that it is estimated that illegal drugs cause about 8000 deaths per year in the USA. This compares to an estimated 130,000 who die every year in America as a result of taking correctly prescribed and correctly administered prescription drugs! I've seen two ways of expressing this. The first shows correctly prescribed and administered drugs as being the third greatest cause of fatality, after heart disease and stroke; the other way shows correctly prescribed and administered prescription drugs as the primary cause of death in America. Statistically, you are 6,500% more likely to die from using these drugs than at the hands of a terrorist! Note: These statistics do not include incorrectly prescribed and wrongly administered prescription drugs.

There would be many great advantages to establishing a chain of government drug stores:-

1. Tobacco and alcohol would be removed from the normal shops. Our children would not come into contact with them.

2. 60% of children in West Yorkshire, where I currently live, have had drugs offered to them in the school playground. If these black market commodities were available in a legal marketplace, that is, if they truly became CONTROLLED SUBSTANCES it would be in no-one's financial interest to push them onto innocents – there would be no profit in it because black-market prices would not apply. Organised crime would lose all interest. The government, though, would be in a position to tax these materials and still sell them at a true market price and the crime rate would plummet. To make an addictive drug illegal is a recipe for disaster. Only a cretin or an establishment hell-bent on maintaining its profits, regardless of the millions of personal disasters that the policy would cause, would come up with such an idea.

3. Users of all drugs would be assured about the purity of the drugs and the hygiene of associated materials (such as needles). Theoretically this would reduce the number of accidental deaths to virtually zero, except, of course, in the case of tobacco. Users could be given proper information at the point of sale rather than being cast adrift by their government which is the current *status quo*.

4. In the case of botanical drugs, these could then become items of 'fair trade' where the growers would receive proper

recompense for their labours. The same farmers would no longer need to deal with criminals.

5. This would remove a great deal of funding to organised crime syndicates.

6. The level of street-crime would plummet. Charging a fair-trade price would mean that the swine who keeps breaking into my car and getting nothing but costing me an arm and a leg in repair bills would be able to afford his habit without interfering in my life.

All this may well seem like a long diversion from the examination of unsaturates we began with but the same kinds of conspiracies apply, just as much, to the universal sale of 'pure vegetable oils'. Indeed, while the European Community attempts to suppress the use of crucial nutrients such as vitamin C and selenium, it SUBSIDISES the production of unsaturated fats and sugar, the two main causes of obesity, heart disease, cancer and type ll diabetes.

My comments about tobacco, above, may seem a long way removed from the discussion of polyunsaturates but there is a clear link between both these substances and lung cancer. The demographics demonstrate that, although many fewer people smoke now than did in the 1930s, and they do not smoke the full tar cigarettes which were popular then, the incidence of lung cancer has risen by a factor of six in the intervening period. This parallels the growth in the use of polyunsaturates and it is now suspected that these oils act as a catalyst for all sorts of cancers.

That said, and I'm sorry a lot of it was negative, lets take a look at some of the exceptional therapeutic properties of the medium-chain fatty acids found in coconut oil. "It is rare in the history of medicine to find substances that have such useful properties and still be without toxicity or even harmful side-effects". So writes Professor Jon J Kabara of Michigan State University.

We have long known that mother's milk has medicinal benefits aside from those conferred on the baby. Prof. Kabara and his colleagues examined three hundred fats over a period of thirty years to find out if there were any which demonstrated the same anti-microbial virtues as mother's milk, palm kernel oil and coconut oil. There were none. He then turned his attention to the medium chain fatty acids and monoglycerides found in these three substances.

According to Prof. Kabara, medium chain fatty acids
1. Have 10% fewer calories than other fats.
2. Are less likely than other fats to be deposited as adipose tissue.
3. Elevate thyroid function.
4. Do not raise cholesterol levels.
5. Do not encourage the growth of tumours (while it is well documented that polyunsaturates do. In animal tests 32% of those fed on corn oil developed cancer of the colon while only 3% of those fed on coconut got the cancer.
6. The monoglycerides in coconut oil are similar to those found in saw palmetto berries. Men over the age of 40 are recommended to take a dietary supplement of this for prostate health. "A dietary approach to healing benign prostate

hypertrophy may be available" (that is the introduction of coconut oil into the diet of the patient). *Many thanks to J J Kabara for the research leading to this information.*

The debate concerning the balance of omega 3s and 6s (so-called *essential fatty acids*) in our diet continues but it seems to me that the balance of saturates to unsaturates is much more important. It may be that one of the major reasons for the growth in the incidence of osteoporosis is that the body needs at least 50% of its fat intake to be saturated in order for calcium to be absorbed into the bones.

According to Dr Joseph Mercola, saturates protect the liver from alcohol and other toxins and omega 3 fats (the ones most people are supposedly short of) "are better retained in the tissues when the diet is rich in saturated fats. The fat around the heart should be highly saturated and it is this reserve which the heart calls upon in times of stress." He goes on to say that scientific evaluation of artery clogs reveals that only 26% is saturated. "The rest is unsaturated of which more than half is polyunsaturated".

I would never have dreamed that there might also be a psychological advantage in consuming saturated oils but a recent study suggests that, while lifestyle changes have lowered the mortality rate from heart disease over the past fifty years, the overall mortality rate remains unchanged. The reason for this is the growth in the incidence of suicide. It would appear that individuals whose saturated fat intake is low are at risk of depression, the severity of this depending on how little of this type of fat is consumed. On a personal note I can comment that, although I've never been prone to depression as such, my mood is considerably better than it was before I ditched the unsaturates.

There is a glimmer of hope for the seed oil producers although, I must admit that, because it's of no interest to me, I've not looked into the economics of it. The internal combustion engine can be adapted to run on this kind of oil instead of petrol. Indeed there are many folk in Britain running their cars on cleaned, used cooking oil. Obviously fuel from an annually renewable source is preferred to fossil fuel. There's a feasibility study for someone!

Since I started passing this article around amongst my friends and clients, many people have asked me what kind of coconut oil they should use. There are basically two types. The first, refined coconut oil, is extracted from copra which is the name given to dried coconut meat. This is often smoke-dried which process imparts a heavy smoke flavour to the oil which is one of the reasons why it has to be refined. The refined product has no flavour or fragrance but, as far as I can tell, it exhibits all the properties of a medium chain fatty acid (as mentioned above). When I first discovered the marvelous properties of coconut oil, the refined product was all I could find and I was very pleased with it indeed as compared to margarine and the unstable unsaturates and polyunsaturates both in terms of the flavour (texture in the mouth might be a better way to express it) and the way it made me feel.

The second product is virgin coconut oil with the organic version of this in the same group. The virgin oil is pressed from the fresh meat of primo coconuts and then filtered. This oil has a delicious coconut flavour which, perhaps unexpectedly, enhances the flavours of most cooked foods. (Seldom does one form the impression that coconut flavour has been added). The virgin oil contains much more lauric acid which is anti-microbial and anti-fungal.

Refined coconut oil is relatively easy to find (health food stores etc) and is relatively inexpensive. The virgin oil is only just beginning to find a foothold in the market place (because of the bad press formerly given to all saturated oils) but if you pester your shopkeeper they should be able to stock it for you.

7

The Old Bazaar in Cairo

Cairo, the capital city of Egypt is situated on the banks of the Nile. One year in the early eighties two momentous things happened there. The first, on 6 October 1981, was the assassination of Anwar Al Sadat or, as the Copts called him 'The Black Ass' (Ane Noir).

The second thing was that I went to live there. I was actually on the beach in a place called Ismailia, when I heard the news of Sadat's assassination. The atmosphere in Egypt changed with one tick of the clock. Before the tick, Egypt had been the most liberal of Arab countries, its people light-hearted and fun-loving despite the tribulations of living in an overcrowded, third world country. After the tick, all entertainment was cancelled. Nothing but the Qur'an was aired on television and radio and the building in which I lived had six armed policemen guarding the door rather than two, one or, sometimes, none. That wasn't exclusively for my benefit. The other occupants of the building were mostly generals, admirals, or dentists, all highly valued personnel.

I'd been in Egypt on holiday the year before but this had done nothing to staunch my appetite for all things Egyptian. I duly rented my place in Morton to my friend Pete Carroll, the writer, packed a couple of bags and set out to meet my destiny in the Land of the Pharaohs (hem hem).

While it had been Anwar Sadat's mistake to let the Hebrews in, it had been to Ramses' great relief that the Hebrews wanted to leave. As far as he was concerned they were a bunch of misfits and no-hopers he was pleased to see the back of. History's like that. It's the guy who writes latest who gets his side of the story heard. Ramses might well have been one of the greatest rulers of all time but, as we commonly receive the story, he's only a foil for Moses – he who went up the mountain and came back down with ten fragments of Hammurabi's Code (which Jews and Christians would contravene throughout history.)

Not that it was only Egypt's Pharaonic past which interested me. The earliest Christian churches and monasteries are to be found in Egypt. I found the atmosphere of these places worthy of Edgar Allan Poe and Ridley Scott and the internal architecture is unique and stunning. I can't comment on the external architecture because I can't remember seeing any of it. Old Cairo is a very close-packed place!

I do recall the exterior of St Michael's, a monastery deep in the desert, in hundreds of square miles of nothing, on the way from Cairo to the Red Sea. It has a featureless and very high stucco wall in which there had not even been a gate or door until the requirement for tourist cash suddenly emerged in the 1970s. Until then the only way in or out was by lift, powered by a donkey. The implication was that, once you were in there, you were in for life.

Much more stunning and unexpected for me was the splendour of the Islamic art and architecture to be found in Cairo and one of the first people I befriended there was the man in charge of Islamic monuments, the guy with the keys!

We picnicked in palaces where no-one had been for years. We drank coffee in the Greer Anderson house (made famous in a James Bond film) with the fountains turned on, as if we were the Pashas normally in residence there. I also got to go inside the medieval city walls, replete with hieroglyphs because the stone had been plundered from the pyramids.

The particular foundation date of Cairo was calculated by astrologers who believed that the rising of Mars would be a particularly auspicious time. And so it was that Mars, God of war, The Conqueror, El Qahira, gave his name to the city. To this day Cairenes do not pronounce the letter qoph (q) at the beginning of words except in two instances, El Qur'an (The Quran) and El Qahira (Cairo).

Of course, I had another mission in Egypt. It is one of the few countries where perfumeries abound, the kinds of places where SOME raw materials are kept. If you're buying patchouli or sweet orange or sandalwood, you're on pretty safe ground if you know something about these items. But if the man in the shop starts talking 'Nefertiti' or 'Queen of the Desert', you're about to spend a lot of money on something that should cost virtually nothing and which has probably been dumped in Egypt by the European perfume industry. Clive James once strutted his stuff in a Cairo perfumerie and ridiculously, considering he was on camera, paid £100.00 for something that should have cost a fiver. It can't have been the BBC then – must have been Channel Four (and I intend no sort of near-miss pun on Chanel 5!)

Most of the perfumers occupy shops in the medieval market area known as 'Khan El Khalili'. There have been aromatic suppliers there since the earliest times of the market, near the spices, many of them concentrated in The Street of the Perfumers or *Attareen.*

Attr means essence in Arabic and gives us the English word *otto* as applied, uniquely, to distilled rose oil. The word *ruh*, spirit or breath, also applies.

My greatest aromatic interest at that time was in recreating *ruthvah*, the so-called 'perfume of immortality', made famous by Aleister Crowley. I say 'made famous by' advisedly because I've never found a reference to it other than in books by or about Crowley.

At that time my enthusiasm for finding the ingredients and making ruthvah overshadowed the ethical implications which now forbid me to make it. Ruthvah is, to put it simply, an animal product.

The perfume of immortality is compounded from musk, ambergris and civet. Musk is extracted from blackish granules about half the size of a piece of maize, found in a surprisingly large pod or external gland at the rear end of the male musk deer. The animal is very small. For all I know it may be the smallest deer on the planet. It is an extremely timid creature which has never been successfully held captive, let alone bred in captivity.

Musk pods consequently have to be taken from hunted animals. Because of the musk deer's timidity and because it lives in the difficult terrain of the Himalayas, hunters shoot any musk deer they see which means that the killing is indiscriminate, females and juveniles being killed in the same numbers as the pod-bearing males.

The species is so endangered that there have, for many years now, been international treaties in place which are supposed to restrict the annual, worldwide use of musk to about 10 kilos, although this is overtly flouted by the French and Far Eastern perfume industries.

In the Qur'an there are many references to perfumes and there is little doubt that the most esteemed perfume in Arabia at that time was musk. (*qv*) Sura (verse) 143 reads 'The Seal of musk. For this let those pant who pant for bliss.'

I was once offered a fresh, whole pod. As its owner unwrapped it from brown paper the smell suddenly became overpowering and I found myself taking a couple of steps backward in shock. It's difficult to imagine how anyone might have thought that if you tincture this stuff in alcohol for at least a year it will have a fixative effect in any perfume to which it is added. There are one or two cities in the Middle East where musk was added to the mortar for the building of defensive walls. I understand that the musk can still be discerned.

Similar remarks apply to the other two ingredients of my quest. Ambergris is a pathological secretion of the sperm whale. These mighty creatures graze on plankton but occasionally they swallow cuttlefish which have very sharp 'beaks'. These can become embedded in the wall of the whale's stomach which must be distressingly painful.

The whale's reaction is to produce a mucous around the site of the injury. It continues to do this until the beak is prised away from the stomach wall. The whale then throws this up and as it contacts the water it hardens and floats away. Lumps of ambergris as big as boulders are occasionally found washed up on beaches, the most famous of which was found by a teenage boy in Aden. The lump of ambergris towered above him. I often wonder if the boy spent the remainder of his life in the opulent style of an Eastern potentate or whether he was palmed off with a lolly and a trip to the cinema.

I own a piece of ambergris (to my shame!) which contains a cuttle-fish beak. The way I came upon it is a tale in itself. Because I was here there and everywhere in terms of perfume suppliers in Cairo, I was able to broker a deal between one of the downtown perfumers and my friend Ali Mohammed Omran who had two shops in the Khan El Khalili, one which the government knew about and on which taxes were paid, and another, more secret salon, exempt from taxation because the government knew nothing of its existence. It was a massive lump of ambergris. I can't remember the weight but Ali paid £3000.00 for it, an incredible sum in a country where a policeman was paid (at that time) £6.00 per month. Ali did all the usual tests before parting with his money. Did it burn? Did it float? etc. Satisfied, he wandered back to the Khan El Khalili and sold the whole lot in £10.00 deals during the course of the same afternoon. My cut was a schnazzy lump of ambergris, (complete with the, now famous, cuttlefish beak) and a parcel of saffron.

Tourists in Egypt are often persuaded to buy a substance referred to as 'amber paste'. The salesmen's story goes that if one smears a little of this filthy stuff on a cigarette and then smokes it, or adds a little to a cup of tea or coffee and drinks it, that one's sexual potency will be up-rated. This, of course, is not true. It was not true even when the paste was formulated on real ambergris.

The Armenian merchant who sold Ali the ambergris used to make the 'genuine' paste himself. Among his clients (urbane folk mostly on the intellectual side of life) it was referred to as 'heart medicine'. When I asked him, naïve to a fault, how this heart medicine was used, he raised a stumpy finger and replied in his very thick accent "You rub it on the gland!".

A more expensive product by far than the paste offered to the tourists in the bazaar, I can see no reason why this product should achieve the desired effect either. As far as boofing up the flagging male libido is concerned, it seems that the more rare, the more expensive and the more bizarre the substance, the more sought after it is likely to be. Rhino horn, tiger teeth, dessicated sea-horse and, indeed, the fabled ruthvah itself are all examples of this.

At the time of this tale I hadn't managed to shake off the tobacco habit and, because it was there and I had plenty of it, I crumbled a gram of ambergris into some tobacco and smoked it. But the last thing I was looking for (at the age of thirty) was an aphrodisiac effect. There is a suspicion amongst some westerners that ambergris has a psychotropic effect. It hasn't, but I felt extraordinarily peaceful for a couple of hours.

The third ingredient of ruthvah is civet, a dark brown, pasty substance which is scraped from the anal pouch of the male, Ethiopian Civet cat. The civets fare rather better than the musk-deer in that they don't have to be killed but the animals are very reluctant captives and I understand that the process of removing the excretion from the gland with a wooden spatula is extremely painful and unpleasant. The animal world should thank the Great Spirit for the availability of Viagra!

I obtained some very old civet from Ali. It was in its original tin caddy and dated 1910, but the years didn't seem to have detracted from its immense odour. In former times civet was containered in impressive looking animal horns sealed with wax.

Perfumers describe civet as having a 'faecal' note. Everyone who puts their nose into my caddy recoils in horror. From infancy we are taught to avoid substances that smell even vaguely like this.

Whoever thought of compounding these three substances? The civet smells like concentrated poo, the musk smells like super-concentrated pet-shop and the ambergris smells like very old books or, perhaps, sun-dried cow-pats.

Each of these substances is highly prized in the making of first class perfumes. A perfume must have an animal note, otherwise it's not much more than a cologne and, where a cologne is intended to be refreshing, a perfume is designed to be a sexual attractant. However, Madame Pretentious would never wear a perfume if she could actually detect any of the animal ingredients which are, consequently, blended into the perfume at below the threshold level. (see Ch. A Rose by Any Other Name).

The ruthvah which Mr Merryweather of Armours compounded for Aleister Crowley was, more than likely, in the form of a paste, similar in consistency to petroleum jelly, but, since it contained nothing but animal product, the notion of threshold level simply didn't come into it. I can only presume that it was applied to the skin in the minutest amounts. It would otherwise have acted as a repellent of all people and creatures (except flies).

There is a fourth animal product which is used in perfumery and I was more than surprised to find it in Egypt. That product

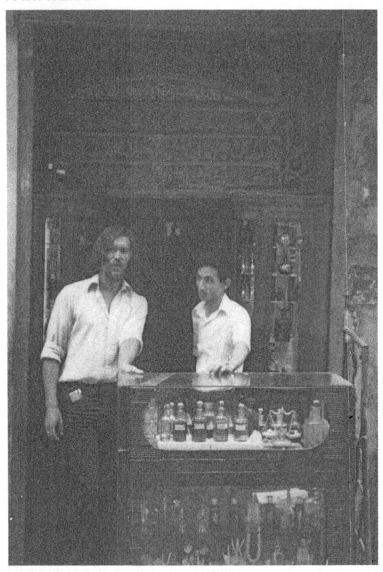

I used to visit Ali Omran as often as I could. He was knowledgeable, witty, and his place in Khan El Khalili, Cairo's Medieval market, was frequented by an immense variety of fascinating individuals.

is castoreum which is the scent gland of the male beaver. The glands come in pairs, as supplied by the hapless beaver, and look like nothing if not like dried human testicles still in the bag. When I asked my Armenian friend if he ever came across these a glint appeared in his eye and he beckoned me to follow him. We left his shop, crossed the road and entered a non-descript building. Inside he showed me two rooms both of which were filled with castoreum pods. It felt to me a little bit like visiting a holocaust museum where one can see piles of hair, much still plaited, still bearing ribbons. The pods must have represented the killing of thousands of beavers. Even when I was using animal products in perfumes I never really found a use for castoreum and I much regretted the killing of so many animals for such a little used ingredient.

In the months during which I was lurking around in the Khan El Khalili I became known amongst the merchants as 'The Dangerous One' because they misinterpreted my interest in perfumery as an interest in how they ran their businesses.

Most of the perfumeries in the bazaar, and there are many of them, have touts working the streets to 'catch' customers. Anyone who's spent time there will be familiar with lines about 'my brothers shop' and 'my friend in Manchester'.

I was having a wander around one day when I was pestered by a boy of twelve or thirteen who was very insistent that I go to his 'brother's perfumery'. Confident that no shops in Khan El Khalili had musk, ambergris or civet, I told him that these were the only items I was interested in.

> *"My brother has these – he has them!"*

> *"I don't want to waste my time.*
> *What if he doesn't have them?"*

> *"You can kill me if he doesn't have them!"*

Game on! I duly followed the young tout for a few minutes and arrived at a shop I'd never been to before.

> *"This boy says I can kill him if you don't have*
> *musk, ambergris and civet."*

The merchant, who was sitting at a desk, looked down without saying anything, opened a few drawers, found what he was looking for and handed it to me – a very large dagger with a curved blade! The boy went white for a moment and then we all had a good laugh about it.

I got to know the merchant, Gamal, very well. Some years later he enabled me to be the first importer of the delicate perfume bottles which are now to be found in shops all over the UK. Despite having a shop in prime-site Khan El Khalili, a nice apartment in Gizeh and a large Mercedes, Gamal is a Bedouin. Totally perplexed at my vegetarianism (it was to be some years before I became vegan) he asked what I might eat if he invited me to dinner. I told him I ate bread, cheese, eggs and that sort of thing.

When dinner was laid out on huge metal trays on the floor, I had three plates, one with a dozen hard boiled eggs, one piled high with rumi, a plastic-like cheese, and a third stacked with *baladi* or country bread, each piece something like a coarse, thick chapatti. Because this was a Bedouin feast there were also many crates of beer which rather made up for the food. I occasionally wonder what Gamal would make of my veganism.

I once walked into Gamal's perfumerie with a bag of netteya I'd managed to find in the spice-market. This is a kind of soft frankincense which can be used as a natural chewing-gum. I was more interested in what it would smell like when it was burned. When I mentioned I'd just got some of this stuff all the guys in the shop said, more or less in unison, "*netteya ya basha!*" with a metaphorical winkle in the eye. It turned out that *netteya* is yet another substance that the Egyptians use to flog the dead horse of a flagging male libido.

It was while I was in Egypt that I began to sell perfumes I'd made myself. My clients were mostly from the British Council or the Embassy. One evening, while I was working on the development of a perfume I started to lose consciousness and had to crawl out onto the balcony for air. The next day, with permission, I tried the compound on someone else with the same result. I kept the formula, quite a complex one, for a few years and then decided to destroy it. I've never recreated the effect and I've never found any reference to such a thing in the literature of perfumery. I would advise anyone with an interest in this anomaly to start with musk *xylol* and *terpineol*, but don't blame me if you go this way!

I mentioned that Gamal helped me to get some hand-blown bottles together. On this occasion I'd made a special trip with Michael, my partner, to do just that. We ended up with about eight hundred bottles which we brought back on the plane! Back at the shop, when we had time to examine the exquisite bottles we'd bought, we discovered the word OSRAM clearly inscribed on two or three of them. The Egyptians don't waste anything.

I'd been having real trouble getting an export license to get the bottles out of Egypt. Even greasing palms wasn't helping and we were working to a time limit. While I was dashing around doing what I could I met a young tour guide at the airport who asked me what my problem was. When I told him of the difficulty I was having he told me to think no more about it. He was actually most interested in introducing me to his father who had been a General in the army but who was now running a trading company.

We duly had a meeting with the General but couldn't muster any interest in the trousers and such that he was hoping to export. Nevertheless, true to his word, the young man got us, and the bottles, out of the country with no problem. He asked us to wear T-shirts when we went to the airport and, despite the fact that our huge box went through the x-ray machine and looked like a box of bubbles, we were not questioned and our box went straight through to the cargo area. Our guide went through with us because, being a tour guide, he had a pass.

When I asked him how he'd got us through so easily he explained that he'd told the customs guys that we were punks, hence the requirement for T-shirts. I looked at him quizzically. "They know that punks are very smelly and don't want to go through their bags", was the only explanation he gave.

It was the General who introduced us to the most exotic perfumer I've ever come across. In the vast, new suburb known as Nasr City, we were taken to what seemed, from the outside, to be a typical Egyptian apartment building. The interior of the man's apartment, though, was a complete surprise. It was like a palace! There were massive chandeliers, exquisitely made. There were superb, gold-leafed chairs and glass cabinets here and there containing the beautiful crystal bottles (up to one litre in size) in which he containered his oil samples.

The man, the General and his partner and Michael and I sat down together round a glass-topped coffee table. Coffees, Pepsis and ashtrays appeared and were put on the table. Then we got to talking turkey and, each time I mentioned an oil I was interested in, a boy rushed off, usually out of the room, and came back a few seconds later bearing one of the enormously expensive bottles, often containing an even more expensive oil.

As our session progressed the table became more and more overcrowded. Nothing was put away. The General and his partner were totally unaware of what was going on and chatted, smoked, reached for their Pepsis and their coffees. I was becoming concerned. By this time there must have been £20,000.00 on the table and these morons weren't even trying to be careful! As it turned out, our party left without having caused any damage.

Michael had been most impressed that the General's partner

had evidently been totally oblivious to the fact that, at one point, he'd had two mosquitos drilling into his face. I was reeling, and reeled for a couple of days, at the oils I'd been sampling. I'd been particularly impressed with the aloewood I'd sampled (see ch Hocus Pocus) but on the table there'd been jasmine, rose, ful, which is similar to jasmine, and many other exotics that I'd never come into contact with before. Michael and I walked the five miles or so back to our hotel, the now-famous Windsor, and arrived there in the small hours of the morning in a cloud of exotic perfume.

I had many adventures in Egypt. One which stands out in my memory doesn't involve aromatics but might entertain anyone with an interest in the place or the period. I've visited the Horus Temple in Edfu several times, partly because of the information about natural medicines carved into the walls. During one visit there was an earthquake while I was in the inner sanctum. The temple is a massive edifice with walls many feet thick. To feel it all moving was a truly awesome experience.

On another occasion I got talking to one of the Bowabs, the men in galabeyas who lurk around looking atmospheric. He asked me if I'd like to see something interesting. When these guys ask you this question they usually want a fiver to show you something you've already seen, but there was something about this man which engaged my enthusiasm. He went from foot to foot until he was sure there was no-one else about, then piled three rickety wooden chairs on top of each other. This enabled us, precariously, to climb into a hole in the wall about ten feet up.

Once we were in the hole the Bowab lit a small candle which revealed a tunnel, running at that height inside the wall. At one point he indicated a hole in the floor of the tunnel which appeared to be bottomless but, having avoided falling down it, there were no further obstacles.

Eventually we came to a tiny room, maybe two metres by one. At this point the Bowab left. I'm not sure how because he left me the candle. I gave my head a metaphorical scratch. The only feature in the room was a recess of a few inches, about the size of a small window. I noted flowers and the remains of incense on the shelf created by the recess. Pretty much by accident my head went partly inside the recess and, suddenly the sound of my breathing was considerably amplified.

On the basis of 'when in Rome' I decided to intone an Ancient Egyptian spinning mantra. With the first phoneme, I knew that an awesome sound could be heard all over the huge temple, both inside and in the courtyards. Some friends of mine were in the outer courtyard, fifty or sixty metres and thousands of tonnes of stone away. They heard the mantra clearly and immediately knew it was Sherwin up to something.

I concluded that this unique acoustic effect would have been used on the occasions when the great unwashed were permitted into the temple, perhaps on one day a year. The priests would have been dressed as Gods with marvellous costumes and masks. When they came to speak, this marvellous effect would have given the impression that the God's voice was shaking the temple and must have had a terrifying impact on the simple folk congregated there.

I got to Edfu, on that occasion, by fallucca, the traditional Nile boat with stupendously tall sail and liftable keel for where there's little depth in the river. A stupendous journey from Aswan it took two days (after I'd spent three days hunting down a *tassrieh,* written permission to travel on the river!).

At one point where the river was wide with desert on each side, I saw a dust-devil, something like a mini tornado, start up in the distance. After watching it for a few seconds I realised, with a sickening feeling in the stomach, that there was a strong possibility that this growing, angry looking thing was heading directly for the boat. I did some quick guess calculations, quite anxious by now to assess the effect of such a thing hitting the enormous sail of the fallucca.

I needn't have bothered. The guy at the tiller, at first unnervingly blase, suddenly braced himself with his back to the side of the boat and his feet on the tiller. As the dust devil hit he became more vocal and started to feverishly offer prayers to Allah, which I didn't find very reassuring. However, his prayers were answered.

The edge of the boat came within an inch of going underwater as the wind slammed into the sail and knocked the boat by 65 degrees or so. My hand, which had been white-knuckle-gripping the side of the boat, got wet. Two days on board was enough for me, especially since a night sleeping on deck meant sharing with the boat's rats, who only emerged at night, and I went on from Edfu to Luxor by train.

On the opposite side of the Nile to Luxor is The Valley of the Nobles in which there is a tomb which has a marvellously acoustic interior. I went there at midday in midsummer, a time when even the flies hardly move, so that I could have a bash at one or two mantras in private. The effect was wonderful, rather like being inside a bell. When I finished singing there was an enthusiastic, solo, round of applause from the entrance. A Japanese tourist had unexpectedly braved the intense heat and I'd not heard him arrive.

There was one extraordinary event, in no way connected with the main subjects of this book, which cannot escape a re-telling. One day I'd taken two English friends who were staying with me to see the Greer Anderson Museum, near the Citadel. Afterwards, we sat down at a street cafe for refreshment and a quick chat before I went to work at the academy.

My attention fell on an amorphous black mass, slightly in shadow at the other side of the road. It moved about a little but I couldn't discern what is was, and we puzzled over it for a couple of minutes. The awful truth dawned as two hands appeared from the centre of the shape. This was a person. The mystery deepened when I realised that the hands were shelling garden peas into a bucket set to one side. Now and then a hand came up to where the mouth must be and put a pea-pod in.

Now I could tell what was going on but it's difficult to believe, even though I saw it myself in daylight without the benefit of alcohol or similar. As the arm moved, a small proportion of the many kilos of flies which were occupying this individual moved enough to give occasional glimpses of part of the face or the filthy galabeya. We watched this playing out for about fifteen minutes before I had to go.

Egyptian Musicians. The women are wearing perfumed wax cones on their heads. As the wax melts down them, it releases its perfume.

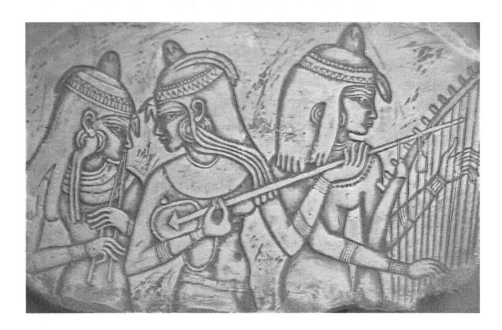

8

Using Essential Oils Therapeutically: Introductory Remarks

Since the mid 1980s, there has been a staggering over-emphasis on what has come to be called *aromatherapy safety data*. Of course there are some oils which are toxic but these are rarely found in the public marketplace. No-one with a commercial interest in these commodities wants to poison the clientele or run the risk of a financial backlash caused by injury.

In more than twenty years of dealing with (literally) thousands of people and hearing of many cases where oils have been abused (infants and adults drinking them neat, for example) I have heard of no cases where permanent problems have been caused. In the early nineties the Poisons Unit at Guy's Hospital considered all essential oils to be potentially fatal because its method of analysis at that time was hopelessly flawed, all essential oils being considered to be chemically the same as turpentine!

The bottom line is that if you use an essential oil within the usual guidelines the chances of an adverse reaction of any sort are astronomical and where an adverse reaction is encountered, all you need to do is stop using that oil and the problem will go away. This is in distinction to allopathic drugs whose side effects can be awesome and permanent, sometimes 'requiring' the introduction of further pharmaceuticals to offset the effects of the first. This leads to the vicious cycle experienced by many, particularly old people, who take twenty or thirty pills for breakfast.

Pregnancy is another case in point. The public is constantly warned about the dangers of using essential oils during pregnancy despite the fact that I've never heard of any pregnancy which suffered because of essential oils. The people who warn about essential oils in pregnancy are often the same ones who prescribe horrendous drugs to expectant mothers and consider these to be safe because they've been through 'clinical' trials. Look at the known side effects of any pharmaceutical drug before you take it because your GP is unlikely to do so. Consider thalidomide, a drug designed to improve fertility which went through clinical trials and then ruined the lives of many mothers (even if it didn't ruin the lives of their children for whom the subsequent abnormalities were 'normal'). Essential oils do not do this.

Herbalism has been with us for much longer than aromatherapy. Has anyone ever seen a safety data index in a herbal? There

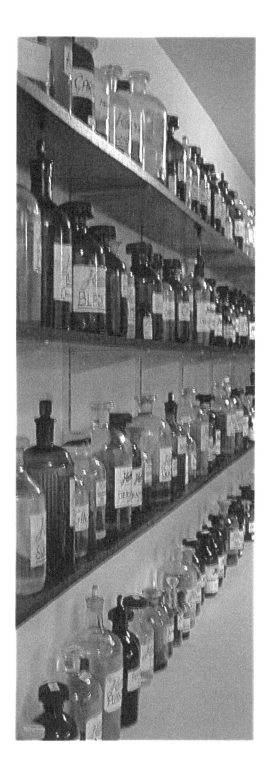

Ray's office at the Hermitage, 2009.

are comparatively few toxins in the plant world and, if you were self-administering herbs, it would be very unlikely that you would be in possession of hemlock or that you would take enough belladonna to cause convulsions. The great poisoners of history usually chose arsenic, puffer fish ovaries or similar.

Consider the current fatuous debate about cannabis. This herb has a track record of three thousand years and no known side-effects except the one that makes people feel contented and pleased. The estimated fatal dose of cannabis is 50,000 times the normal therapeutic dose, an amount which it would be impossible to take. Contrast this with aspirin, one of the West's favourite pharmaceuticals, whose fatal dose is 25 times the normal therapeutic dose and whose administration to under 16s may cause Reye's syndrome.

If you were depressive, which would you choose?:- A botanical drug with no side effects and with a real cost of virtually nothing.

A pharmaceutical drug (eg Prozac) with a list of possible side effects as long as your arm the first of which is **possible liver failure** and which costs more than £1.00 per dose?

Did you ever hear of a Prozac user being counseled about the safety data of that drug? Of course not. Valium was introduced to the medical profession as a crisis treatment never to be used for more than three weeks, yet there are so many Valium addicts in society that they are a positive menace. Driving under the influence of Valium is even more crazy than driving under the influence of drink yet, despite the development of tests to check the level of cannabis in the blood (which does not affect skills such as driving so long as it is not used in conjunction with tobacco) there seem to be no plans to test drivers for allopathic medicines which severely affect the mentative processes.

Drug companies are well-known for playing both sides against the middle so that, for example, pharmaceutical companies' trade reps will often encourage doctors to prescribe 'outside the box'. That is, they will, for example, encourage the prescription of drugs for children which are only intended for adults but a concerned parent phoning the company will be told "Oh no, we don't recommend its use for children." The company makes the money, the GP hopes to get the child's parents off his back and no-one is any the wiser until the child starts to suffer. In the event of adverse reactions (which are, contrary to popular opinion, extremely common) the GP will probably prescribe further pharmaceuticals which will, more than likely, cause further problems. The pharmaceutical company is laughing up its sleeve because it's making yet more money and the GPs happy because he can be seen to be doing something (useless though that might be in a final analysis).

At the time of writing, the pharmaceutical companies are seeking to establish a complete stitch-up in terms of nutritional supplements. Consider this. The EU, under enormous pressure from the pharmaceutical companies, intends to ban the sale of selenium. If the UK still received its grain from Canada, which has selenium content in the soil which is passed into the grain which in turn is consumed by humans who, in their turn, absorb the selenium, there would be no problem. However, since the formation of the EU, nearly all the UK's grain has come from Europe. There is virtually no selenium in European soil. Outcome – selenium depletion. Since selenium is one of our most effective anti-oxidants (*ie* anti-cancer nutrients) one can only view the intention to deny it to the public as extremely sinister indeed.

Selenium is only one of many hundreds of examples but I've chosen it because I can use it as a simple illustration. A recent study (2003) concludes that men whose selenium levels are depleted are at four to five times the risk of developing prostate cancer. Given that prostate cancer is, next to lung cancer, the cancer from which men are most likely to suffer, the intention to ban the supplement cannot be considered to be benign. Infantile asthma may be on the rise as a result of the absence of selenium in the diet.

As I mentioned above, this is an illustration. I could list many of these. The selenium is not an isolated case. Who wants to cure cancer? Not the pharmaceutical companies! It's in their interest that as many people as possible contract cancer so that they can prolong it to make even more money. This is why the drugs companies detest the idea of people taking the responsibility for their own health by carefully selecting what they eat and drink and by using natural medicines such as essential oils and herbs. Because so many people in the western world are waking up to this, the only recourse for the drugs boys is to make the materials difficult or impossible to obtain. Consequently, expecting real information on health from drugs companies is comparable to asking Adolf Hitler for help on the ethics of running a prison.

Back to the plot! Of course, in any healing discipline one needs to know if the client is suffering from any condition which would be worsened by the introduction of a particular therapeutic agent. But consider this; the health problems of the twentieth and twenty-first centuries are largely to do with the human organism coming into contact with molecules never before encountered in the history of human evolution. The incidence of carcinogens in particular has been increasing exponentially since the beginning of the industrial revolution but there are molecules in many allopathic medicines which the human organism has never before encountered and which, in consequence, the body is unsure how to deal with.

Often a 'modern' molecule is the cue for disease whether it's encountered as a pollutant or a medicine. In stark contrast to this, humans and their forebears have developed alongside plant molecules for hundreds of millions of years and, with the exception of plant toxins which are very rare, have developed an organic understanding of those molecules. It is this organic understanding which more or less guarantees that disciplines such as aromatherapy and herbalism can be practiced with impunity. Of course the dosages have to be reasonable and possible contra-indications have to be checked out but other than that, as I contended at the beginning of these remarks, aromatherapy safety-data has been over emphasised.

Companies selling essential oils are forbidden by law to say anything in print about the therapeutic nature of the oils they sell. For many firms, all that remains is safety data and a great song and dance is made about it. The aromatherapy schools join in the dance because safety data, in contradistinction to everything else about aromatherapy, can be learned parrot fashion. It's easy and virtually spurious.

Over the last hundred years humanity has had a mighty trick played against it. We were all led up the path that says **science explains everything** or **science has an answer for every problem we suffer from**. This attitude is virtually the same as the one that says 'The Earth is supported on the back of a giant tortoise'. Science and technology have caused more health problems than they have relieved and aromatherapy, of all the alternative health disciplines, gives us the opportunity to sidestep the simplistic, mechanistic approach of allopathic medicine into a realm where instinct, intuition and imagination are considered useful adjuncts to the knowledge of healing rather than barriers against it.

I referred earlier to clinical trials. As far as I can make out there seem to be two kinds of these, the first kind being independently funded (these are few and far between) and the second kind being funded by food and pharmaceutical companies. We could all be forgiven for feeling re-assured that our breakfast cereal or the medicine we are taking has been fully assessed for effectiveness and safety if clinical trials were the exacting procedures we were brought up to believe they are. Unfortunately they are not. Many so-called double-blind clinical trials are neither double-blind nor clinical in a sense that would satisfy those of us who might be looking for objective evidence rather than a sales pitch and a document to satisfy the regulatory authorities. In many cases the regulatory authorities seem to work hand in glove with manufacturers rather than protecting the interest of the consumer.

In the case of food, for example, it's taken many years for the Food Standards Agency to consider banning the use of the hydrogenated oils which are routinely used to bulk out a vast array of foods, despite the fact that we've known for many years that trans fats are negatively nutritional. Negatively nutritional? Indeed, these lab-created semi-solid fats remove nutrients from the human body rather than making a contribution.

In the case of drugs trials, manufacturers often tailor the placebo to suit the trial. For example, vaccine trials never seem to use an innocuous placebo. They usually contain what it pleases the drugs companies to call 'serum' which means, in short, everything that goes into the vaccine except for the bacterium itself. Where you might have expected that the placebo group was dosed with nothing at all, those individuals get the mercury and formaldehyde which is used in the complete vaccine to depress the activity of the bacterium.

Follow up studies are short and incomplete because they only include a small percentage of the individuals in the trial. This example is not isolated – it is, unfortunately, typical and puts the whole notion of pharmaceutical intervention into disrepute. Because clinical studies are fudged, not only as just described but in other ways too, it is impossible to claim that immunisation works because there is NO SCIENTIFIC EVIDENCE that it does. In this respect the pharmacetical companies have shot themselves in the feet. Looking in from the outside at the 'results' obtained is very interesting indeed. There was recently a measles outbreak in London which affected thirty children. Of the thirty, thirteen had received the triple vaccine known as MMR.

How must the parents of those thirteen have felt when they realised that they'd taken the considerable risk of having three diseases plus mercury and formaldehyde injected directly into their child's bloodstream, without any of the promised benefit of the vaccine being conferred? (As an aside to this, it seems bizarre that an authority looking for 100% take-up of the MMR permitted the inclusion in the vaccine of porcine gelatine, automatically ruling out Jews, Muslims, vegetarians and vegans).

It is entirely hypocritical that a country which makes such a huge song and dance about so-called illegal drugs should depend, as it does, for a large slice of its GDP on pharmaceuticals which have been improperly trialled.

Cannabis received its bad press because, on a level field, it would take something like 40% of the pharmaceuticals market (a staggering amount of money). Such losses cannot be countenanced by an industry based on mass production and mass marketing. I expect that the impact of legalising cannabis for therapeutic reasons would rock the stock-markets in a way that they've never rocked before!

To a lesser extent these remarks apply to essential oils in the same way as they do to cannabis. Oils are cheaper to use than pharmaceutical drugs and perform some medicinal functions much more efficiently than synthetics. They therefore represent a threat to the pharmaceuticals industry in whose interest it is to emphasise the potential dangers of aromatherapy. The market does not want patients undergoing chemotherapy to use cannabis as an anti-nausea treatment because the real cost of such a treatment would be about 20p as opposed to allopathic anti-nausea treatment which would cost about £300.00. The market doesn't want parents getting rid of their kids' verrucae using lemon oil at an approximate real cost of £1.00 when it can burn out verrucae and earn itself £100.00.

A friend of mine was once prescribed a systemic fungicide for an aggravation under the fingernail. As a consequence he lost his sense of taste for almost three months and also lost a couple of stones in weight as a result. He didn't, however, lose the fungal aggravation until I recommended he dose his finger with tea tree oil. One dose later the problem had gone completely and there were no side effects in the wake of the 'cure'. **The cost of this treatment was so small as to be incalculable.** That's a horrifying prospect for the market.

Furthermore, using a systemic fungicide for this kind of problem is as ridiculous as a farmer would be if he sprayed a whole field with weed killer just to get rid of a few dandelions in the corner. The dandelions get killed but so does the crop. If the crop isn't killed it's sold to you complete with its dusting of poison. (It's worth mentioning that when my friend next went to see his GP – this time with his eyes a little more open

– he noticed the name of the company who manufacture the fungicide which had caused all the trouble on the wall-clock, the calendar and the desk-pad!)

Be sensible with essential oils. Use good housekeeping procedures. Keep bottles etc clean. Keep your oils away from children. Check that the oils you would like to use on a client are not contra-indicated. Then let your imagination go. Aromatherapy is not a systematised discipline and is hindered by the allopathic approach. My friends finger was helped by tea tree oil but lavender, thyme, orange, ylang or geranium might well have done the job just as efficiently. Aromatherapy is an art more than a science and the longer it remains an art rather than being 'pseudo-scienced' the longer it will be of great benefit to us.

Paracelsus said that everything is toxic. What he meant was that toxicity is a dose-dependent state and that we can kill ourselves with the most innocuous substances (eg water) if we overdo it with them. As a rule of thumb, the essential oils to be found on the High Street have GRAS status – that is, they are Generally Recognised As Safe. Do your background research but don't be afraid to experiment. With essential oils you can retake the responsibility for your own health that was stolen by the health marketeers. Eat good food, take regular exercise, smell sweet!

The above is written from the aromatherapy viewpoint and, as a consequence, allopathic medicines take a thrashing. From a more general viewpoint it's reasonable to suggest that all disciplines of healing whether they be patriarchal and mechanistic (so-called orthodox medicine), or matriarchal and chaotic (aromatherapy and other holistic disciplines) have their strengths in particular areas of healing and for particular individuals. In short, horses for courses. Acute appendicitis is not best treated with aromatherapy – infections are not necessarily best treated with antibiotics.

Please don't take the above remarks to be an encouragement to ignore the safety data. We all need to know as much as we can about not poisoning ourselves and our friends.

9

Monographs
On My Favourite Oils

There is a slight overlap of information between this section and the remainder of the book. This has been done intentionally so that there are no major omissions in the monographs.

Essential Oils and Absolutes: Methods of Extraction

Essential oils are not all the same. Each has its own fragrance, properties and peculiarities. Each behaves in its own characteristic way. Perhaps it boils at a particularly high temperature (useful as a fixative), or has a high antiseptic value or perhaps it contains a rare therapeutic agent such as azulene (in chamomile). Whatever the reason for its uniqueness no essential oil is the same as any other and this includes oils distilled from plants of the same species in different places or at different times. For these reasons, anyone who wants to understand essential oils must understand the individual characteristics of all the oils he/she uses. However, there are some generalisations that can be made about essential oils, as follows:-

ESSENTIAL OIL – DEFINITION: Essential oil is distilled

or pressed from plant parts. The product so obtained may or may not be further refined depending on circumstances. Regardless of its origin an essential oil is volatile which means that it will evaporate into the air. Essential oils dissolve in alcohol and in fixed oils but not in water.

The word *essential* is misused in English to imply importance or necessity when, in fact, it is the adjective formed from the noun essence. Other languages are more specific. Arabic, for instance, uses the word *ruh* which means spirit or breath, implying that the fragrant oil is the very life of the plant from which it was obtained.

The most common misunderstanding about essential oils is that they are produced by steeping the plant parts in a fixed oil. It is possible to produce a mildly fragrant oil in this way but nothing so powerful, intense and persistent as an essential oil or an absolute.

ABSOLUTE – DEFINITION An oil produced by solvent extraction. Quality jasmin oil is only extracted by this method. Rose oil is produced both as an otto (by distillation) and as an absolute. The two products differ considerably largely because phenyl ethyl alcohol (one of the constituents responsible for the fragrance) is soluble in water and, therefore, hardly present at all in the otto. There used to be concern that some of the solvent remained in the oil. These days though, extraction by carbon dioxide or hexane is extremely sophisticated and the possibility of solvent residue is not an issue.

Absolutes dissolve in alcohol and fixed oil but not in water.

FIXED OIL – DEFINITION

Vegetable oil (usually cold pressed), *eg* sweet almond which does not evaporate at all. Fixed oils have no fragrance value but find extensive use in aromatherapy and cosmetics.

EXPRESSION

The simplest extraction process, expression is most suitable for fruits whose oil, contained within the peel, is liberated when the tiny capsules which contain it are burst. When the fruit has been separated the peel is put into presses and the oil is squeezed out. With the oil come water and impurities which must be removed before the oil can be used. Fruit oils can also be distilled. In the case of bergamot and lemon, for example, the distilled product contains no furocoumarins and this makes for a safer oil for both therapist and patient.

DISTILLATION

The most common extraction process. In its simplest form distillation entails immersing plant parts in water, boiling the mass and collecting the liquid which accumulates from the vapour produced. Although this method may be considered crude it remains the most effective way of extracting delicate oils such as rose and orange blossom since the highest temperature that can be reached is 100c.

Using steam distillation quite high temperatures can be reached, especially under pressure. Superheated steam is passed through the plant parts and then condensed whereupon the oil separates from the water. High temperatures liberate aromatic substances which might otherwise be difficult to extract.

SOLVENT EXTRACTION

The traditional way to capture the fragrance of delicate flowers (*enfleurage*) uses warm or cold lard as a solvent. Flowers are placed on *chassis*, wooden framed sheets of glass onto which lard has been spread. Over the ensuing hours (or days!) the lard absorbs the aromatic constituents of the flowers. The flowers are then removed and the *chassis* is recharged with fresh flowers, this process being repeated until the lard is saturated. The resulting waxy and fragrant substance, *the pommade*, is then *subjected* to alcohol to wash out the oil it contains. The alcohol can then be evaporated off leaving *the absolute from pommade*.

The *enfleurage* process is seldom used today but perfumers look back to the old fashioned product with a certain nostalgia since it allowed enzymatic decomposition to take place and this resulted in some exciting peculiarities of odour. As the name implies, solvent extraction causes substances such as petroleum ether to pass through the prepared plant parts. The solvent is then evaporated off leaving a mixture of waxes and oil. This is called *the concrete*. After the removal of the waxes there remains the highly fragrant, intensely strong substance known as *the absolute*.

Perfumery and aromatherapy are related disciplines and to understand one of them it is an advantage to know at least something of the other. The aromatherapist needs to know how to blend therapeutic oils for the maximum effect and yet achieve a product which is also pleasing in its fragrance. The perfumer needs to be aware of the physiological and psychological effects of the oils in order to induce in the person who wears the product a feeling of well-being and specialness.

10

Using Aromatherapy products at home

Essential oils and absolutes are safe for administration in the home provided that a few simple rules are observed:-

Oils should not be ingested unless a competent practitioner has recommended this course of action.

Avoid contact with the eyes and mucous membranes.

When adding essential oils to the bathwater don't use more than four drops. Some books recommend higher dosages than this – please ignore them.

Essential oils should not be self-administered by pregnant women, especially during the first sixteen weeks of pregnancy. Thereafter, consult a practitioner who will tell you which oils are safe in your case.

Do not administer essential oils to babies. All treatments for infants should be in consultation with your doctor/practitioner.

Although there is a general recommendation that oils should not be applied undiluted to the skin, this does not apply to the tiny (less than one drop) amounts which might be used for 'routine' injuries.

When using essential oils, wash your hands before as well as after visiting the lavatory.

Store oils in a dark place at low room temperature away from foodstuffs and out of the reach of children and pets.

Massage oil should consist of 3% essential oil(s) to 97% fractionated coconut oil or other fixed oil. Most treatments are dose-dependent and making a blend stronger does not mean that this will make it more effective. As a rule of thumb, ten drops of essential oil(s) should be dissolved in 16ml of fractionated (or virgin) coconut oil. If you're using a blend for the first time, test it on a small area of skin before doing a complete massage.

Do not use oils in any form while you are engaged in strenuous exercise or while you are in a sauna, steam room or other humid environment, since high humidity effectively doubles the quantity of oil absorbed.

Do not use seed oils or so called 'pure vegetable oils' as carriers. They are unstable and contain solvents.

11

The Monographs

ALOEWOOD

NAME Aloewood, agar wood, bird wood, eagle wood, el
oudh, kaju lakka

BOTANICAL NAME Aquilaria Agallocha

YIELD I am unable to ascertain the yield but it must be very
small indeed, annual output of the whole planet amounting
to only a few kilos.

SOURCE East India (Mysore, now Karnataka), Vietnam

COLOUR light to dark yellow/gold

METHOD OF EXTRACTION steam distillation of the
fungus infected wood. Only mature trees (more than fifty years
old) are used for oil production, the less esteemed parts being
used for making (very expensive) incense. When it has been

cut, the wood is placed in water. The infected parts are heavier than water and these are saved for distillation. This selection procedure gives rise to the Chinese name for a very similar wood, 'Fragrance sinking under water'.

SAFETY DATA Not known, but the oil has been used as a perfume for centuries with no known ill effects.

PERFUMERY USES Aloewood is one of the few essential oils to have an animal note which makes it invaluable especially in perfumes which, for whatever reason, do not contain any of the classic animal notes. Used by itself it is a wonderful, masculine perfume much prized in the Gulf States where the price can be anything up to £500.00 for 10ml on good batches.

ATTRIBUTION Jupiter? Archangel Michael

ADDITIONAL INFORMATION Aloewood has been a prized material since Ancient Egyptian times. It is very likely that the aloes referred to in the Biblical references to incense is aloewood and not the juice of the common aloe as is generally presumed. Get hold of a gram or so and enjoy it - it's almost addictive.

BASIL OIL
– EXOTIC OR SWEET? THAT IS THE QUESTION.

In the late 1980s there arose a concern that basil oil was potentially irritant and possibly carcinogenic. This led those of us who were interested in its qualities to look in some detail at the *material medica*.

Aromatherapy books often recommend that members of the

public should buy the most expensive oils available (presumably because the authors think little of their readers' intelligence!). There are several reasons why this might not represent the best advice foremost among these reasons being pertinent to the basil question. There are two basic chemotypes of basil. The first is exotic basil (so called) which is sought after for perfumery and flavouring and is the more expensive of the two types. The level of methyl chavicol, the component which alerted suspicion about basil oil, is far too high – typically 70 – 90%. The level of eugenol, another suspect is also high.

For these reasons the therapist should use only the linalool type of sweet basil where the linalool represents about 40% of the mass and methyl chavicol is present at only about 23%. This oil is safe within the usual guidelines but should be avoided, as should most essential oils, during pregnancy.

BERGAMOT

NAME Bergamot

BOTANICAL NAME Citrus Bergamia

SOURCE extracted from the fresh peel of the fruits of the tree which grows principally in Calabria - the fruits are collected in November and December

COLOUR green

SPECIFIC GRAVITY around 0.884

MAJOR CHEMICAL CONSTITUENTS chlorophyll, linalyl acetate, linalol, terpenes, sesquiterpenes, bergaptene

(except in the bergaptene free material)

METHODS OF EXTRACTION The oil is pressed from the peel. Any oil remaining after this process is distilled out but the distilled product is less highly esteemed.

SAFETY DATA Known to sensitize the skin of some individuals. It is perhaps best to assume that all the fruit oils are photosensitising. Bergaptene free bergamot may be considered safe within the normal therapeutic guidelines.

THERAPEUTIC USES Bergamot is largely used to bring about elevation of mood.

PERFUMERY USES The best oil comes from ripe fruits which produce an oil of high ester value. Used mostly in colognes and fresh or green perfume types.

ADDITIONAL INFORMATION Bergamot is best known as the flavouring in Earl Grey's tea. Dodgy tea bags can be converted into something drinkable by the addition of one drop of already diluted oil.

BLACK PEPPER

NAME Black Pepper

BOTANICAL NAME Piper Nigrum YIELD 1 - 2.3%

SOURCE Southern India, Philippines, West Indies.

COLOUR colourless to yellowish

MAJOR CHEMICAL CONSTITUENTS phellandrine, dipentene, piperine, a pinene, limonene, terpinolene, terpinen-

4-ol, b-carophyllene, d-cadinene.

METHOD OF EXTRACTION Steam distillation of the dried, crushed, unripe berries with the pericarp removed.

SAFETY DATA To be used sparingly in cases where kidney disorder is present. Use 1.5% dilution in fevers, 3% dilution in other cases except where prolonged treatment is necessary, in which case use 1.5% in order to avoid possible local irritation.

THERAPEUTIC USES This oil introduces heat and is beneficial where, for example, the mobility of a joint may be enhanced. Traditionally black pepper oil has been used in cases of male sexual dysfunction.

PERFUMERY USES Used in fancy perfumes and soap perfumes. Toner in carnation compounds (along with clovebud oil). A small amount of black pepper oil added to an aromatherapy blend may 'boof' the product and make it more interesting.

ATTRIBUTION Mars

ADDITIONAL INFORMATION The oil is first mentioned by Salah El Din (Saladin). Its first mention in connection with medicine is in *Dispenatorum Noricum* (1589).

CEDARWOOD OILS

NAME Cedarwood

BOTANICAL NAME Juniperus Virginiana (USA), Cedrus Atlantica (Africa)   **YIELD** 2.4 - 4.5%

SPECIFIC GRAVITY 0.945 - 0.960

COLOUR Pale yellow to almost colourless

MAJOR CHEMICAL CONSTITUENTS Cedrol, cedrenol, pseudo-cedrol.

METHOD OF EXTRACTION Distillation of the chipped wood.

SAFETY DATA Most emphatically, cedarwood oil should not be taken by mouth and should not be used during pregnancy.

PERFUMERY USES Cedar gives a warmth and depth to many types of perfumes and 'after-shaves'. More particularly it is used to tone violet and white rose creations.

ATTRIBUTION Jupiter

ADDITIONAL INFORMATION Perhaps not suprisingly, the inhalation of the vapour of cedarwood oil imparts a violet odour to the urine. Other oils, rose or sandal for example, maintain their own fragrance identity when passing out of the body, whether they pass in the urine (sandalwood), feaces (rose) or gas!(rose).

Occasionally oil from the East African cedar, juniperus procera, appears on the market. It is similarly priced but of rather finer odour than the American. All types of cedarwood have been used extensively to ward off insects and rodents. Cigar boxes used to be made of cedarwood for this reason. Great buildings (including Solomon's temple) used cedar not only because it continues to exhale its fragrance for hundreds of years but also because it is less liable to attack by insects. The Ancient Egyptians, who prized cedarwood so highly that they annexed Lebanon where the finest trees grew, oiled their papyri with its oil to protect them for posterity.

An oil extracted from cedar leaf is occasionally offered under the name thuja which name refers to cedarwood as a species. It has a bright, dynamic fragrance but is toxic and should not be used in aromatherapy. Thuja (Gr) means 'to fumigate' or 'to sacrifice' which indicates that the Greeks valued cedarwood chippings as an incense. The notions of incense and sacrifice were closely linked in the mind of the Ancients, the smoke carrying the supplications of priests and others to the heavens. The word 'fumigate' comes from the Latin *fumare* - to smoke and is the basis of our word perfume (*per fumum* - through smoke). The etymology of words connected with the subject of smell is a tangled trail always leading us back to man's first experience in controlling the nature of his olfactory environment - incense. That first experience probably happened at the same time as the discovery of fire since, in the case of labdanum, cedar, sandal, pine and many others, all man had to do was to throw it on the fire.

Cedarwood forms part of the base-note complexes of a variety of perfumes.

Examples follow:-

ORIENTAL NOTE   Woodhue by Fabergé

FOUGERE NOTE   Flor de Blason by Myrurgia

FLORAL NOTE   Pavlova by Payot

GREEN NOTE   Mademoiselle Ricci by Ricci

CHAMOMILES

NAME Roman Chamomile, German (blue) Chamomile.

BOTANICAL NAMES Anthemis Nobilis (Roman), Matricaria Chamomilla (German).

SOURCE Western Europe and the Americas (Roman), Germany, Hungary, Egypt (German).

MAJOR CHEMICAL CONSTITUENTS (Roman) esters of butyric acid, azulene, chamazulene, coumarin. (German) azulene, chamazulene. Although azulene becomes green, or even brown, quite readily, this is not an indication that the oil has become useless as an anti-inflammatory. The colour of the oils, Roman or German, is not an indication of quality or otherwise.

CONGEALMENT POINT Crystallisation begins at 15 degrees C. The oil is solid at 15 degrees C.

COLOUR Both oils are ostensibly blue (keeping in mind the remarks made above).

METHOD OF EXTRACTION Steam distillation of the dried flowers.

SAFETY DATA Safe within the normal guidelines.

THERAPEUTIC USES It is very important that the following information quoted from Jean Valnet's excellent book *The Practice of Aromatherapy*, be circulated as widely as possible amongst health care professionals.

"The bacteriostatic effect of azulene is produced at a concentration of 1 part per 2000 parts against *staphylococcus aureus*, *haemolytic streptococcus* and *proteus vulgaris* in particular. Infected wounds have been healed using concentrations of from 1 part in 85,000 to 1 part in 170,000." Uses for impetigo and MRSA need to be fully investigated but it looks like we should forget all about the tea tree in these cases!

PERFUMERY USES Both oils are used as toners in floral compositions. The blue is also used in oriental perfumes, chypre and fougere types.

ATTRIBUTION Sun (attributed by the priests of Ancient Egypt.)

ADDITIONAL INFORMATION Oil of chamomile is first mentioned in the price ordinance for Frankfurt in the year 1587. It was originally believed that the oil was blue because of some reaction between the distillate and the copper distillation vessels.

However, this was proved to be untrue when a blue oil was produced using glass equipment. The colour is now known to result from the presence of azulene, formerly called coeruleine. The common name of both types is derived from the Greek *kamai melon* meaning ground apple because of the fruity scent of the crushed flower. The Spanish common name *manzanilla* has the same meaning.

There is, to the present day, an argument about whether or not German chamomile is a true member of the chamomile family since it does not have a number of the physical characteristics required. True chamomile or not it contains much more of the precious azulene than the Roman type. A more important point to note is that most aromatherapy suppliers offer a product confusingly referred to as Moroccan chamomile which definitely does not belong to the chamomile family. This oil is *ormensis multicaulis* and, while it may have a slightly sedative action it should not be substituted for German or Roman chamomile and may safely be considered to be a spurious oil. During the nineteenth century, chamomile oil was often distilled over lemon peel to increase the yield. References to lemon-chamomile may also be safely regarded as spurious.

To confuse the picture a little more, German (blue) chamomile is largely grown and distilled in Egypt.

A NOTE ON CINNAMON OIL

Just in case you haven't used cinnamon leaf before, please be aware that it needs to be substantially diluted before use and carefully patch tested on the client/patient. Cinnamon does not damage the skin but it has a warming effect which can be experienced as a burning sensation by some individuals. At the right level of concentration the warming effect soothes pulled, tired or aching muscles.

CLARY SAGE

NAME Clary Sage

BOTANICAL NAME Salvea Sclarea

YIELD 0.117%

SOURCE Southern France, Hungary, Russia

SPECIFIC GRAVITY 0.907 - 0.928

MAJOR CHEMICAL CONSTITUENT linalyl acetate, traces of thujone as in common sage oil

COLOUR Colourless to pale yellow

METHOD OF EXTRACTION Steam distillation of the flowers. A lesser product is prepared from the whole herb and this finds use as a perfume fixative. This product is sometimes referred to as vegetable amber and is not used therapeutically.

SAFETY DATA Alcohol should not be consumed after a treatment with clary sage as this may lead to nightmares, although, I must say, that's more a serving suggestion than a proscription. After treatment it is best to wait for an hour or more before driving or operating machinery. Following a number of scare-reports in the newspapers which claimed clary sage oil to be narcotic I spent some hours sniffing a bottle of fine quality French clary with 'disappointing' results.

THERAPEUTIC USES Clary is usually the first resort for 'female problems', especially period pain. It is considered to be a uterine tonic. It has a powerful relaxing effect.

PERFUMERY USES Most artificial perfumes are improved by the inclusion of a small amount of clary sage, particularly amber and chypre types. It helps to 'round' products which might otherwise be harsh although this quality might not be immediately apparent, at least a month's maturation time being necessary. Clary also finds use in the manufacture of colognes to which it gives warmth and sweetness.

ATTRIBUTION Culpeper suggests the moon. I would suggest Venus.

ADDITIONAL INFORMATION Clary sage was introduced into English cultivation in 1562. The name clary evolved from the Latin clarus meaning 'clear' and the herb has been called 'cleareye' or eyebright because of its supposed effectiveness in clearing foreign bodies from the eye. The herb is also known as 'muscatel sage' since it was first used commercially by wine merchants who infused it with elderflowers and added the liquid thereby obtained to the Rhein wines which we know as muscatels. It is also used in the preparation of vermouth.

Although the pure oil has little instant appeal, a dilution of clary sage might well be described as being warming and exotic. Usually described as being similar to lavender oil, presumably because of its high linalyl acetate content (between 38% and 72% depending on growing conditions, maturity of the plants etc.), I would suggest that its closest fragrance counterpart is rose otto and, indeed, it is often substituted for rose otto in perfumes and preparations for which rose is considered too expensive. It is also used as a fragrance ingredient in its own right. Examples follow:-

CHYPRE NOTE   Parure by Guerlain

ALDEHYDE NOTE   Opéra by Coryse Salomé

FLORAL NOTE   Raffinée by Houbigant

GREEN NOTE   Quant by Quant

HANDY TIP While the price of Hungarian and Russian clary sage is attractive the oil is not. Buy these and you're likely to be disappointed. The French material is, in every way, superior.

EUCALYPTUS

NAME Eucalyptus

BOTANICAL NAME Eucalyptus Globulus, occasionally E. Radiata

YIELD up to 3%

SOURCE Australia, Spain, USA, Italy, Algeria. The Blue Gum tree from the leaves of which the oil is obtained can attain a height of 350ft. Other types of eucalyptus can reach as much as 450ft in height which makes them the tallest tree in the world.

SPECIFIC GRAVITY 0.910-0.930.

MAJOR CHEMICAL CONSTITUENTS eucalyptol, d-pinene, terpineol, iso-borneol, camphene, ethyl alcohol, aromadendrene and phellandrine. The last two constituents mentioned oxidise to form ozone.

METHOD OF EXTRACTION Distillation of the fresh leaves.

SAFETY DATA Safe within the normal guidelines. High dosage can irritate the kidneys (by which it is excreted). See end note 'Handy Tip'.

THERAPEUTIC USES We're all familiar with the decongestant properties of this oil. It also finds use in joint-mobility preparations.

PERFUMERY USES E Globulus is used extensively in the manufacture of perfumes for soaps and detergents. Other eucalyptus oils (see additional info) are used in quality perfumes according to their nature.

ATTRIBUTION No valid attribution.

ADDITIONAL INFORMATION Oil of eucalyptus was first mentioned in 1790 but it was not until 1854 that Bosisto, who had previously experimented with distilling the dried leaves, opened a distillery in Australia. Eucalyptus trees have been planted in marshy places prone to malaria (eg Campagna, near Rome). The beneficial influence exerted by the tree in this circumstance probably has more to do with its draining effect on the land than with the influence of the leaves' aromatic principle on the air.

The name derives from the small membrane which covers the flower bud in its early stages [Gr eucalyptos = covered].

There are more than three hundred species of eucalyptus. Of these the oils of the following are particularly worthy of mention:-
E Citriodora   a lemon type fragrance
E Macarthuri a rose type fragrance
E Staigeriana a verbena type fragrance

My earliest memory of eucalyptus oil is, as a small boy in the fifties, having road tar removed from my clothes with it. It is a solvent for tarry substances and was used a great deal for the removal of stains until chemical stain removers became available. (Some years after writing the above, an ugly road tar stain appeared on our computer-room carpet. Not heeding my advice, the cleaner tried all sorts of 'tried and tested methods' which did not address the problem at all. One wipe with a tissue containing a little eucalyptus and the stain was gone!)

HANDY TIP Because there is some evidence (scant though it might be) that eucalyptus is not suitable for treating infants and young children, wise therapists often substitute RAVENSARA aka rich man's eucalyptus with good results.

A Note on Fixed Oils

Fixed oils and creams have a limited shelf life. Oils such as avocado can go ropey (long strings of material accreting in the mass) within three months of purchase. If the supplier has had the oil in stock for two months before you get it, the life of the oil is virtually finished! Other oils simply go rancid and, in most cases, there are no off-notes to inform you of this. Rancid oils are comparable to hydrogenated oils, that is, they have negative nutritional value and negative therapeutic value. Pigs and rats, better informed by their nervous systems than humans, will have nothing to do with rancid or hydrogenated oils and we don't want you to have anything to do with them either. Recent research shows a strong connection between trans-fats **and Alzheimer's Disease and other very serious illnesses.** Most supply companies specialize in sweet almond oil because, they claim, it is the aromatherapy oil *par excellence*. If you're going to use this make sure that it is lead-free. The best course of action is to use fractionated coconut oil which, unlike the polyunsaturated oils, is stable.

Of the unsaturated and polyunsaturated oils, the most stable (in terms of both therapy and nutrition) are the oils which have been available for centuries such as almond and olive. **Seed oils are unstable at room temperature, unstable at cooking temperatures and unstable as soon as they have been absorbed by the body**

The healthiest option for cooking with is coconut oil, a saturated (and therefore stable fat) which the body uses for energy and which is not stored as fat like the long chain fatty acids. Coconut oil is a known booster of thyroid function (see Ch. The Fats of Life) whereas seed oils are thyroid antagonists and may be the main contributing factor to the current trend towards obesity.

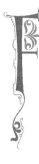

FRANKINCENSE

NAME Frankincense, Olibanum

BOTANICAL NAME Boswellia Carterii

SOURCE Southern coast of Arabia, East Africa

YIELD 8%

SPECIFIC GRAVITY 0.875 - 0.894

MAJOR CONSTITUENTS a-pinene, camphene, dipentene, para-epinene, olibanol

COLOUR Clear to light yellow

METHOD OF EXTRACTION Steam distillation

SAFETY DATA   Safe within the normal therapeutic guidelines.

THERAPEUTIC USES Frankincense is a brilliant pulmonary antiseptic and can be used to advantage where stress is a factor of the illness.

PERFUMERY USES Used to 'pre-fix' alcohol - about 1ml frankincense to 1 litre ethanol which should be left to mature for about one month before use. This process 'softens' the alcohol and helps to create a more natural fragrance. Frankincense finds much use in heavy, oriental types of perfume and in many mens' fragrances.

ATTRIBUTION Sun

ADDITIONAL INFORMATION No aromatic commodity has a more interesting history than frankincense. To begin with the names:-

Frankincense is derived from the Old French meaning 'real incense'. Olibanum is a corruption through the classical languages of the Arabic luban which strictly means 'gum' but, in practice, is always applied to this commodity. (see Ch. Hocus Pocus for more on frankincense.)

GERANIUM OIL

NAME Geranium

BOTANICAL NAME Pelargoneum Graveolens

YIELD 0.02%

SOURCE Extracted from the leaves of the plant belonging to the N.O. Geraniaceae which grows principally around the Mediterranean although it is a native of Southern Africa. The volatile oil was first extracted in 1819.

SPECIFIC GRAVITY 0.888 - 0.897

MAJOR CHEMICAL CONSTITUENTS pinene, geraniol, citronellol, linalol, terpineol, menthol

COLOUR green

METHOD OF EXTRACTION steam distillation

SAFETY DATA Safe when used within normal therapeutic guidelines.

THERAPEUTIC USES I use geranium for cold sores. At the first hint, blast it with neat geranium. If you catch it early enough you'll forget you were about to get a cold sore. The oil is also useful in cases of chicken pox, shingles and gout.

PERFUMERY USES Widely used in floral bouquets, artificial rose ottos and quality soap perfumes.

ATTRIBUTION Aries (Crowley), Venus (Culpeper)

ADDITIONAL INFORMATION Not that this is a universally applicable piece of information but anglers sometimes add oil of geranium to their groundbait since this appears to attract fish. There's an interesting line of research for someone.

Although geranium oil is used in feminine perfumes, eg Flora Danica by Swank and Ivoire by Balmain, it finds much more extensive use in the production of male perfumes, or after shaves so called. Examples follow:

GREEN NOTE	Jovan Grass Oil by Jovan Monsieur Lanvin by Lanvin
CITRUS NOTE	Happy by Clinique Napoleon by Juper
LAVENDER NOTE	Pino Sylvestre by Vidal
SPICE NOTE	Cacharel pour L'Homme Old Spice by Shulton

FOUGERE NOTE   Jordache Man by Jordache
                                    Wild Country by Avon

HANDY TIP Although Egyptian geranium oil is a little more expensive than the Chinese material it goes much further.

GINGER

NAME Ginger

BOTANICAL NAME Zingiber Officinale Roscoe

YIELD 2 – 3%

SOURCE Native to India but cultivated in Japan and, more recently, the West Indies.

SPECIFIC GRAVITY 0.875 – 0.885

MAJOR CHEMICAL CONSTITUENTS citral, methyl heptenone, nonyl aldehyde, linalool, d-borneol, gingerin, gingerol, gingerone and zingiberol (probably the main odorant).

COLOUR Pale yellow to amber depending on age.

METHOD OF EXTRACTION Steam distillation of the dried rhizomes.

SAFETY DATA Use in low concentration to avoid possible local irritation.

THERAPEUTIC USES Use in cases where gentle warmth may be appropriate (painful/tired muscles, joint mobility, sexual dysfunction.

PERFUMERY USES Because of its high boiling point ginger

is very useful in fixative compounds. It is used as a toner or warmer in herbaceous creations.

An exotic and warming massage oil (the olfactory equivalent of mulled wine) can be made as follows:-

7 drops clary sage, 5 drops ginger, 3 drops benzoin, 5 drops sweet orange, 5 drops ylang ylang grade 1, in 60ml of fractionated coconut oil.

ATTRIBUTION Sun

ADDITIONAL INFORMATION Ginger should not be confused with snakeroot which is also known as *wild ginger*. First mentioned in the spice ordinance of Copenhagen in 1672, the name is derived from the Sanskrit *Sanjabib*.

GRAPEFRUIT

NAME Grapefruit

BOTANICAL NAME Citrus Paradisi [hybrid]

SOURCE Florida, California, West Indies, Southern Asia

YIELD 0.05 - 0.1%

SPECIFIC GRAVITY 0.860

MAJOR CHEMICAL CONSTITUENTS limonene, cadinene, neral, geraniol, citronellal, paradisiol, furocoumarins

COLOUR Florida grapefruit [var. Duncan] is pink(ish) and is often marketed as 'Grapefruit [pink]'. Other types are yellow/green

METHOD OF EXTRACTION the oil is cold pressed from

the peel. See Bergamot which describes this process.

SAFETY DATA Perhaps the safest of all the fruit oils, nevertheless grapefruit should not be administered to babies and infants. Although grapefruit contains fourocoumarins (cf bergamot and its bergaptene), grapefruit does not exhibit the phototoxicity associated with other fruit oils. This is presumed to be because of a quenching effect of one or more of the oils other constituents.

THERAPEUTIC USES Grapefruit oil has a ph very similar to the skin. Careful use of this oil may help with digestive problems.

PERFUMERY USES Used as the basis of fruity accords grapefruit also provides a fresh top-note useful in colognes.

ATTRIBUTION Sun [?]

ADDITIONAL INFORMATION All types of grapefruit oil oxidise relatively quickly. If you're likely to have it in stock for more than three months it's an idea to take up the head space in the bottle with small glass beads or some other inert material.

JASMIN

NAME Jasmin Absolute

BOTANICAL NAMES Jasminum Officinale, Jasminium Grandiflorum. The latter prefers very warm climates.

YIELD 0.1% (hence the high price!)

SOURCE France, Morocco, Egypt, Algeria, Turkey, India.

SPECIFIC GRAVITY 0.920 - 1.015

MAJOR CHEMICAL CONSTITUENTS benzyl acetate, jasmone, linalool, linalyl acetate, methyl anthranilate, indol. Indol seems to be produced in the flowers mostly after they have been picked and its presence increases the longer they are left before processing. More than 1% of indol renders the oil too pungent for use in fine perfumes and for this reason the flowers, which are picked at night when their perfume is strongest, are processed almost immediately as soon as they are picked.

COLOUR Golden to dark brown.

METHODS OF EXTRACTION Enfleurage. Distillation and solvent extraction have all been tried at some time. Distillation is really too coarse a process for such a delicate perfume. Enfleurage, arguably the best method of extraction has largely been superseded by the more cost effective solvent extraction process.

SAFETY DATA Safe within the normal therapeutic guidelines. Some therapists note that they get headaches when they work with jasmin, possibly because of its benzyl acetate content. There is no reason connected with safety data why dilutions of less than 3% should be used but, because of the incredible strength of the absolute, a 1% dilution is more than adequate. In itself this would reduce the risk of headache in those who are prone. Ensure good ventilation.

PERFUMERY USES One of the most important materials used in perfumery. It is the most used floral oil because its indol content imparts an animal note impression below threshold levels.

Examples follow:-

Youth Dew by Estè Lauder, Shalimar by Guerlain, Shocking by Schiaparelli, Opium by Yves St Laurent.

ATTRIBUTION Moon, Diana

ADDITIONAL INFORMATION Ernest Parry, *Cyclopaedia of Perfumery*, (1925) gives a (perhaps apocryphal) story concerning the introduction of jasmin into Italy which is quoted here in full.

> *"One of the early Dukes of Tuscany was the first owner in Italy of a (jasmin) plant, and as he wished to retain it as a novelty, he forbade his gardener to give away any cuttings of it. The gardener, however, disobeyed his orders and gave his mistress a bunch of the flowers as a birthday offering. She was so pleased with the perfume that she struck some of the branches, and by careful cultivation produced large quantities of flowers which she sold to such advantage that she amassed a great fortune and married the gardener".*

Gethsemane, the garden in which Christ is supposed to have spent the last hours before his arrest, may well have been a jasmin garden, Gethsemane being a corruption of the old name Jessamine. If true it would have been a perfect place for the profound meditations we are told took place there.

JUNIPERBERRY

NAME Juniperberry

BOTANICAL NAME Juniperus Communis

YIELD 0.2 - 2%

SOURCE Mediterranean countries

SPECIFIC GRAVITY 0.867 - 0.875

MAJOR CHEMICAL CONSTITUENTS terp-ineol, a-pinene, camphene, cadinene

COLOUR colourless to slightly greenish

METHOD OF EXTRACTION Steam distillation of the dried, ripe berries.

SAFETY DATA Juniperberry is less toxic than most essential oils and is safe under the normal therapeutic guidelines.

THERAPEUTIC USES Use wherever a diuretic might be needed. I have used this oil with some success to subdue the pain arising from an enlarged prostate.

PERFUMERY USES Used as a toner, mostly in masculine fragrances but also, to an extent, in herb/spice complexes for feminine perfumes.

ATTRIBUTION Ishtar/Inanna/Kepra

ADDITIONAL INFORMATION This oil has been used for two hundred years in medicines (especially for dropsy). However, the history of the plant and berries as a fumigant and incense ingredient stretch back to Ancient Egypt where the berries were one of the ingredients of the notable incense

'Kyphi' which was burned by the priests of Heliopolis in sacrifice to Kep-Ra, the midnight Sun. A number of formulae for this incense have been discovered.

The following is as good an example as any. The product should be soft and sticky.

Example of Kyphi incense:
pine resin , wine, galangal root, rush, juniperberries,
broom, mastic, grapes, honey

Kyphi, because of the inclusion of liquids, is better burned on a hot metal plate rather than charcoals. Not exclusively an incense it was also used in poultice form for ulcers etc and may also have been consumed.

A commodity called 'juniper oil' (note the absence of 'berry') is offered by many essential oil companies. Juniper oil (so-called) is a turpentine-like substance distilled from the twigs and leaves of juniperus communis. It costs about one third the price of the true commodity and should not be used in therapies.

The principal use of juniperberry oil in commerce is as a flavouring, particularly for gin. Another 'juniper oil', consisting of little more than terpenes, the flavour chemicals having been removed, is also offered on the market. This spurious oil, like the one mentioned above, finds little application in perfumery and none in aromatherapy. If in doubt, ask your stockist. If your stockist doesn't know, buy your oils elsewhere.

True juniperberry oil oxidises very quickly and this leads to the formation of insoluble particles. Keep head space in containers to a minimum and store in optimum conditions.

HANDY TIP juniperberry carries away excess fluid from the body. It also carries away toxins, particularly sodium, from muscle tissue.

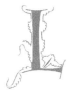

LAVENDER OIL

NAME Lavender

BOTANICAL NAME Lavendula Augustifolium (Officinalis)

YIELD 1.4-1.6%

SOURCE Mediterranean countries, especially France.

SPECIFIC GRAVITY 0.885 - 0.895.

MAJOR CHEMICAL CONSTITUENTS l-linalyl acetate (30 - 45%), esters of butyric acid, propionic acid, valerianic acid. Linalol is present as an ester and in the free state. Geranyl acetate, geraniol, ethyl amyl ketone (which largely determines the characteristic fragrance of the oil).

COLOUR Yellow to yellow-green. Rectified lavender oil (not recommended) is colourless.

FLASH POINT 71 degrees C.

METHOD OF EXTRACTION Steam distillation of the freshly cut flowers.

SAFETY DATA Safe within the usual guidelines. One of the least toxic oils.

ATTRIBUTION Mercury

PERFUMERY USES Lavender oil is mostly used in toilet waters and soaps although it needs to be skillfully compounded with other oils to be of any great value. Of these other oils, geranium, bergamot, rosemary, thyme and patchouli are the most useful.

ADDITIONAL INFORMATION Think of lavender and quite naturally you think of England. During Cromwell's 'Commonwealth' the use of perfume was banned (along with maypole dancing, secular music etc). Many large houses of the time had their own still rooms and continued to distil lavender oil, a simple product which was evidently not classed as a perfume by the authorities.

Lavender is often classified according to its content of linalyl acetate, its principal ester. Lavender oil BP contains at least 39% - other oils might be described as 40/42% or similar. Ester values of 50% have been recorded but these oils are not sought after by therapists.

The finest oils are distilled from plants grown at an altitude of about 1500m above sea level although standard (reasonably priced) lavender will perform all therapeutic actions required of it.

HANDY TIP Lavender oil is a first-aid kit in a bottle. It has the same antiseptic value as phenol.

LEMON OIL

NAME Lemon

BOTANICAL NAME Citrus Limonum

YIELD 0.6 - 0.8%

SOURCE Mediterranean countries especially Sicily and Calabria; Brazil, USA, Argentina, Israel.

SPECIFIC GRAVITY 0.858 - 0.861

MAJOR CHEMICAL CONSTITUENTS citral, citronellal, d-limonene, methyl heptenone, phellandrine, terpineol, linalyi acetate, geranyl acetate, camphene. Like some other citrus oils, lemon contains waxlike substances which may come out of solution following a change in background temperature. Lemon oils with the terpenes removed do not do this but are not recommended for therapeutic use.

COLOUR yellow

METHODS OF EXTRACTION Lemon oil is available as either expressed or distilled material. The old-fashioned method of extraction by hand is quoted here from *Hayle White's Materia Medica* (1929). "The workman holds in his left hand a medium sized sponge, smaller ones being placed between the fingers, or a large sponge is suspended over a pail by means of a stick driven through it. With the right hand he takes a piece of peel and squeezes it in such a way as to break the oil glands and discharge their contents on the sponges. When sufficient has accumulated the sponges are pressed; the liquid thus obtained separates on standing into a lower watery stratum and an upper, clear oily layer which can be poured off. The oil this obtained is filtered off and exported in coppers of varying sizes."

SAFETY DATA May sensitize the skin - best presumed to be photosensitizing. Use the distilled oil since this contains none of the hazardous furocoumarins which are responsible for photosensitization. Maximum two drops in bathwater - do not use on the face or other sensitive areas such as the inner thigh.

THERAPEUTIC USES Gets rid of warts and verrucas (on hands and feet – elsewhere try sweet marjoram oil). Lemons, and consequently lemon oil, may stimulate the production of T-lymphocytes.

ATTRIBUTION Sun?

ADDITIONAL INFORMATION Lemon oil is much used as a flavouring agent. The flavour seems much stronger than the odour so err on the side of caution. Lemon oil discourages fleas.

LIME OIL

NAME Lime oil

BOTANICAL NAME Citrus Aurantifolia

SOURCE Cuba, Mexico, Florida, Italy, West Indies.

SPECIFIC GRAVITY at 29 degrees. 0.873 - 0.882.

MAJOR CHEMICAL CONSTITUENTS citral, linalyl acetate, limonene, cymene, coumarins [in the distilled oil only], linalol.

COLOUR expressed oil - pale yellow, distilled oil - clear.

METHODS OF EXTRACTION lime oil is extracted both by expression and by steam distillation.

SAFETY DATA Only the distilled oil should be used therapeutically. The expressed oil is photosensitizing in the same way as bergamot from which the bergaptene has not been removed.

PERFUMERY USES The expressed oil is preferred in perfumery preparations. It adds freshness, particularly to floral accords.

ADDITIONAL INFORMATION The expressed oil throws down a considerable yellow deposit on standing. The distilled oil does not do this. Some sources suggest that lime oil helps to cope with sadness.

NEROLI

NAME Neroli, Orange Blossom

BOTANICAL NAME Citrus Aurantium

YIELD 0.8 - 1.23%

SOURCE It may be that the bitter orange tree, the flowers of which are distilled to produce neroli, was originally native to Southern China. It was introduced into Europe and North Africa by the Arabs and now grows all around the Mediterranean.

SPECIFIC GRAVITY 0.872 - 0.887

MAJOR CHEMICAL CONSTITUENTS dipentene, pinene, camphene, linalol, geraniol, methyl anthranilate, d-nerolidol.

COLOUR yellowish but brownish red if exposed to light for some time.

METHOD OF EXTRACTION Although the enffleurage process is still occasionally used, distillation is the usual method of extraction.

SAFETY DATA Safe when used within the normal therapeutic guidelines. It is non-irritant and may be used where inflammation is present. The pure, undiluted oil has a stimulant effect on the nervous system and, consequently, may cause headaches.

THERAPEUTIC USES Mostly used to settle the emotions, some claim that neroli helps thread-veins to disappear.

PERFUMERY USES Used extensively in colognes when it is likely to be blended with oils such as bergamot, lavender, lemon, rosemary and petitgrain, neroli is a constituent of the fresh top notes of the following perfumes:-

Mitsouko by Guerlain, Crepe de Chine by Millot, Aphrodisia by Fabergé and Chypre by Coty.

ATTRIBUTION No traditional attribution. I would suggest Jupiter since the golden apples referred to in the myth of Juno may have been oranges.

ADDITIONAL INFORMATION There are many apocryphal stories which account for the name of this oil. That it was Nero's favourite perfume and therefore named after him is, I think, unlikely since there is no evidence to suggest that the orange (bitter or sweet) was available to the Romans at that time. More likely is that the oil was used for perfuming gloves by the wife of Flavio Orsini, Prince of Neroli in about 1680. The distillation of the oil was first described in 1580.

ORANGE OIL [SWEET]

NAME Sweet Orange

BOTANICAL NAME Citrus Aurantium [var. Dulcis]

SOURCE Brazil, USA, Israel, West Indies, Mediterranean countries.

YIELD 0.3 - 0.5%

SPECIFIC GRAVITY 0.848 - 0.852

MAJOR CHEMICAL CONSTITUENTS limonene, linalol, terpineol, citral, citronellal, methyl anthranilate, nonyl alcohol, decyl alcohol.

COLOUR Pale to orange. The presence of a waxlike, non-volatile substance can cause haziness in the oil especially after a change in background temperature.

METHOD OF EXTRACTION Cold pressing of the peel.

SAFETY DATA Best presumed to be slightly irritating. Use low dosage in massage and bath preparations.

ATTRIBUTION Sun

ADDITIONAL INFORMATION Because of the irritation which may be caused to the skin (as with most citrus oils) orange is best used to neutralize the air. Evaporated particles may take some hours to fall to the ground, during the whole of which time they are active, and their antigenic properties continue to function even on the surfaces to which they fall. Orange oil deters fleas and cuts through grease. Orange oil is used extensively as a flavouring. Add a few drops to pancakes and chocolate sauces.

HANDY TIP Sweet orange oil is mildly antiseptic. Use it to wipe down surfaces etc where contagion is present.

PATCHOULI OIL

NAME Patchouli

BOTANICAL NAME Pogestomon Patchouli

YIELD 3%

SOURCE India, Indonesia, China, the Chinese oil being totally inferior

SPECIFIC GRAVITY 0.970 - 0.995

COLOUR dark brown, sometimes with a green tinge.

MAJOR CHEMICAL CONSTITUENTS patchouli alcohol (formerly called patchouli camphor), cinnamic aldehyde, benzaldehyde, eugenol, patchouline.

METHODS OF EXTRACTION The best oil is extracted by direct steam distillation, 240K of the predried herb taking about 24 hours to process. A lesser product is extracted using volatile solvents.

SAFETY DATA Safe when used within the normal therapeutic guidelines.

PERFUMERY USES Patchouli is the fixative par excellence

for heavy perfumes and is employed in traces for the same reason in some rose bouquets. It blends well with most other oils and only one other oil, namely vetivert, has a deeper note.

ATTRIBUTION No traditional attribution. I would suggest Earth or Pan.

ADDITIONAL INFORMATION Patchouli oil was first imported into the UK as part of a counterfeiting operation. During Victorian times Indian shawls imported into this country made very good prices and although it was possible to manufacture similar shawls here the genuine item could be easily identified by its smell. When the eager forgers realized that the characteristic smell was caused by the patchouli leaves in which the genuine shawls were packed and shipped it became the matter of a moment to add a few drops of patchouli oil to the forgeries and the illusion was complete. This led to the first wave of popularity of patchouli as a perfume in the 1860s which was probably only just rivalled by its popularity in the 1960s during which period it received the nick-name 'hippy-juice'. It is one of the few essential oils which improves on ageing.

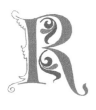

RAVENSARA

NAME Ravensara

BOTANICAL NAME Ravensara Aromatica

COLOUR Clear liquid

CHEMICAL CONSTITUENTS cineol, alpha-terpineol.

COUNTRY OF ORIGIN Madagascar

SAFETY DATA Much safer (in terms of historical safety data) than eucalyptus globulus. Since it is used for conditions where eucalyptus might otherwise be the choice, ravensara is extremely useful, especially in the treatment of infants who are most at risk from eucalyptus.

THERAPEUTIC USES 'Ravensara is of particular value because it is extremely well tolerated, whether inhaled or applied topically. Its mellowness is on a par with true lavender. Its tolerability and anti-viral action make it the essence of choice for the treatment of influenza. It is a central nervous system tonic and its resulting uplifting qualities make it very useful during the acute stages of the 'flu'. May be helpful for insomnia.' Quoted from the excellent book *Medical Aromatherapy* by Kurt Schnaubelt, published by Frog Ltd.

ADDITIONAL INFORMATION There is virtually no information in print about this oil which is why we have chosen to quote Kurt Schnaubelt's comments on the therapeutic nature of ravensara. At one time it was known as 'rich man's eucalyptus' because there was so little known about how useful it was. Ravensara is destined to take a high profile place in aromatherapy along with lavender and tea tree.

ROSE ABSOLUTE
NAME Rose Absolute

BOTANICAL NAME Rosa Damascena

YIELD 0.02 – 0.05%

SOURCE France, Morocco.

SPECIFIC GRAVITY 0.9686 at 20 degrees C.

FLASH POINT 102 degrees C.

MAJOR CHEMICAL CONSTITUENTS phenyl ethyl alcohol, geraniol, nerol, citronellol.

COLOUR red-brown

METHOD OF EXTRACTION by volatile solvent.

SAFETY DATA One of the least toxic oils.

THERAPEUTIC USES Some types of eczema respond to treatment with this oil. Its foremost use seems to be as an abdominal and lower back massage component for the period immediately before childbirth.

PERFUMERY USES Although otto of roses is largely considered superior to the absolute (well, it is three times the price!) phenyl ethyl alcohol, one of the main odorants of the flowers, tends to be present in the absolute to a much greater degree since it is not dissolved away in distillation water. This gives the absolute a more 'nature-identical' perfume.

ATTRIBUTION Venus

ADDITIONAL INFORMATION Poucher observes a) "that no two flowers emit the same fragrance"; b) "that different flowers from the same plant have never exactly the same perfume." It takes 40,000 flowers to make one ounce (about 30mls) of the oil.

ROSE OTTO
NAME Rose Otto

BOTANICAL NAME Rose Damascena

YIELD 0.02 – 0.05%

SOURCE Turkey, Bulgaria

SPECIFIC GRAVITY 0.855 – 0.870 at 20 degrees C.

CONGEALMENT POINT The most highly esteemed rose otto, Bulgarian, congeals at 17 – 21 degrees C. It needs only gentle heat from the hand to become liquid again.

MAJOR CHEMICAL CONSTITUENTS geraniol, l-citronellol, phenyl ethyl alcohol.

COLOUR Light yellow, sometimes with a greenish tinge.

METHOD OF EXTRACTION Steam distillation of the flowers.

SAFETY DATA Safe when used within the normal therapeutic guidelines. Rose otto is, perhaps, the least toxic of all the oils used therapeutically.

THERAPEUTIC USES Some types of eczema respond very well to treatment with rose otto. Use about 5% dilution.

PERFUMERY USES Mostly used in fine fragrances, rose otto is also used extensively as a flavouring (*eg* Turkish Delight). In the Middle East and elsewhere, those who can afford it add rose otto to the drinking water. I never managed to acquire a taste for this but I guess it disinfected the water well enough.

ATTRIBUTION Venus

ADDITIONAL INFORMATION Although it is quite

possible that rose otto was produced long before the birth of Christ, the first definite mention of it was made by Geronimo Rossi in 1574. An earlier work, *The Almanac of Harib* (961 AD), mentions the most suitable time for the production of rose water but the first 'official' appearance of distilled rose oil is in the tax ordinance of Worms for the year 1582.

Of the seven thousand cultivated varieties of roses, *rosa damascena*, because of its hardiness and prolific yield of flowers, is the supreme variety for oil production. It does not occur wild. A 10ml bottle of rose otto contains the product of 20,000 flowers.

ROSEMARY

NAME Rosemary

BOTANICAL NAME Rosemarinus Officinalis

YIELD 1.4 – 1.7%

SOURCE Mediterranean countries, especially Tunisia and Spain.

SPECIFIC GRAVITY 0.900 – 0.920

MAJOR CHEMICAL CONSTITUENTS paracymene, pinene, camphene, cineol, camphor, borneol, lineol.

COLOUR colourless to greenish yellow.

METHOD OF EXTRACTION The cut twigs are allowed to dry in the sun for about eight days. The leaves are then stripped off and steam distilled.

SAFETY DATA For a long time rosemary oil was considered to be contra-indicated in epilepsy. Recent research at Manchester University and elsewhere, however, suggests that regular massage with low concentrations (less than 1%) reduces the frequency of fits in epileptic patients. This matter considered, rosemary oil is safe at normal therapeutic concentrations.

THERAPEUTIC USES This oil finds use in a variety of applications including joint mobility (in rheumatic cases etc.), hair loss, the treatment of head-lice and conditioning of the hair.

PERFUMERY USES Used extensively in herbal creations.

ATTRIBUTION Robert Tisserand gives Sun. I would suggest (obviously for quite different reasons) Moon.

ADDITIONAL INFORMATION Distillation of rosemary oil was first described by Arnoldus Villanovus in the thirteenth century. He distilled rosemary and turpentine together. A similar product known as Hungary water was popular as a perfume and rejuvenator for the next three hundred years. Because Spanish rosemary oil is subject to adulteration and because the Tunisian chemotype imparts an odour of rosemary (rather than rosemary modified with eucalyptus) I always use the Tunisian material.

ROSEWOOD

NAME Rosewood

BOTANICAL NAME Aniba Rosaeodora

YIELD 0.8 – 1.6%

SOURCE Amazon rainforest, Mexico.

SPECIFIC GRAVITY 0.91 – 0.95

FLASH POINT 74 degrees C.

MAJOR CHEMICAL CONSTITUENTS lialol (up to 90%) terpineol, nerol, geraniol.

COLOUR clear to yellowish

METHOD OF EXTRACTION steam distillation of the chipped wood.

SAFETY DATA Safe within the normal guidelines.

THERAPEUTIC USES A calming influence. Use it wherever linalool might be a good influence. Antibacterial, sedative, deodorant. Use in refreshing foot-baths along with peppermint and lavender; in cosmetics for dry skin; in massage for loss of appetite.

PERFUMERY USES Used extensively in fine perfumes and colognes.

Examples follow:- Femme by Rochas, Shalom by J Muller, Ciao by Houbigant, Scheherazade by Desprez.

ATTRIBUTION Venus (?)

ADDITIONAL INFORMATION Rosewood seldom appears in standard texts on aromatherapy and perfumery. Consequently there is little information available which is a shame because it is an inexpensive, pleasantly scented oil. It is a good oil to evaporate at meal times because it covers the smell of cooking without suppressing the appetite like some of the floral and herbal oils. Yes, it comes from rainforest but the trees are not felled for their oil and it would be a criminal waste not take the oil when the tree is already down. At one time anglers used rose otto to flavour their ground-bait. Nowadays geranium, rosewood and aniseed are preferred.

SANDALWOOD
(EAST INDIA AND AUSTRALIA)

NAME Sandalwood (East Indian)

BOTANICAL NAME Santalum Album

YIELD 4-6%

SPECIFIC GRAVITY 0.973-0.985

COLOUR Pale yellow

SOURCE mountainous districts of Mysore in Southern India.

METHOD OF EXTRACTION Steam distillation of the chipped or powdered heartwood and roots. Although sandalwood has often been recommended as an oral treatment (see *A Modern Herbal* by Mrs M Grieve) it is most safely used in massage treatments, poultices, bath oils and evaporators.

PERFUMERY USES Excellent fixative. Used in violet and cassie creations. Blends well with most other oils and is especially useful in sumptuous 'oriental' perfume types.

ADDITIONAL INFORMATION Although the *H & R Guide to Fragrance Ingredients* cites sandalwood oil as one of the "...most expensive raw materials available to the perfumer it must be said that there are many essential oils which are far more costly and much less versatile. With the exception of aloewood oil (which is very expensive indeed) there is no other essence which gives the same voluptuous warmth as sandalwood.

The production of the oil is scrupulously controlled by the government of Mysore, the very best oil being 'agmarked' or approved by the Ministry of Agriculture. Only the heartwood of mature trees (aprox 30 yrs) is used and current reports from Mysore suggest that the use of sandalwood for carving and furniture making is to be curtailed in order to ensure a sufficiency of trees for future oil extraction.

The oil is present to some degree in all parts of the wood and is responsible for the formation of the heartwood. It is not secreted by the wood. This distinguishes it from other woods such as guaiacum and sanders whose heartwoods are formed through the action of resin which is secreted especially when the bark and outer wood are damaged. Sandalwood as a building material was much esteemed in Asia because of its resistance to attack by insects. One of the effects of the oil which I have observed at first hand is its efficacy in warding off mosquitos and other aggravating critters encountered in the East.

Perhaps because it does not smell of flowers and does not contain the fresh and green top notes associated with them, sandalwood has long had a reputation as an aphrodisiac. It is an intimate perfume, in distinction to most other essential oils, largely because of its very slow rate of evaporation, which means that one has to be quite close to smell it at all (except in the case of its being evaporated in which case it can be quite pervasive).

It may be that its aphrodisiac reputation arises from its inclusion (as the active ingredient) in traditional medicines for impotence, most of which are topical lotions, or, more probably, because its perfume is faintly animal/non-floral or, as more descriptive sources have expressed it, 'Naughty!'

East Indian sandalwood oil forms part of the fixative/base-note complex in many and various commercial perfumes regardless of perfume type as the following examples demonstrate:-

GREEN NOTE	Chanel 19; Panache by Nerval.
FRESH FLORAL NOTE	Anais Anais by Cacharel; Lumière by Rochas
SWEET FLORAL NOTE	Ginseng by Jovan; L'Origan by Coty
ALDEHYDE NOTE	Chamade by Guerlain; Moonwind by Avon
ORIENTAL NOTE	Opium by St Laurent; Amun by 4711

When I was asked recently to create a fragrance to be evaporated during the practice of Hatha Yoga I came up with the following simple formula:-

6ml sandalwood, 1ml benzoin, 13 drops clary sage, 5 drops ginger.

This can also be diluted for use as a perfume, massage

oil or anointing oil.

A splendid incense whose fragrance is almost identical to the blended essences can be made by adding a gloop of benzoin and a few drops of clary and ginger to powdered sandalwood.

This is best done in a mortar and pestle in which case the powder and liquids can be easily 'creamed' together, rather like making a cake.

Sandalwood powder takes up an unexpected amount of oil before it becomes sticky. Use just enough of the liquid ingredients for the product to be reasonably dry and burn it on a charcoal disk or hot metal tray.

The price of East Indian sandalwood oil always goes up and never comes down. During my time in the world of aromatics, sandalwood has been totally unavailable on a couple of occasions. These occasions were both connected with the deaths of Ghandis, Indira and, some years later, her son. Such enormous quantities of sandalwood were burned during the periods of mourning that no sandalwood was let out into the world at large and we had to go without.

TEA TREE

NAME   Tea Tree

BOTANICAL NAME   Melaleuca Alternifolia

YIELD   0.33%

SOURCE   Australia (with best oils from the Bungawalbyn area).

SPECIFIC GRAVITY   0.90 – 0.92

FLASH POINT 57 degrees C.

MAJOR CHEMICAL CONSTITUENTS   terpinen-4-ol (should be between 35 and 40% or you've got a 'cosmetic' (*ie* useless!) grade, cumene, a-pinene, para-cymene, limonene, cineol, g-terpinene, a-terpineol.

COLOUR pale to colourless

METHOD OF EXTRACTION   Steam distillation of leaves and branchlets.

SAFETY DATA People with sensitive skin should use less than 3% dilutions and might benefit from blending the oil with sweet almond or similar before adding it to the bathwater.

THERAPEUTIC INFORMATION   Tea tree kills things. Efficiently. Use it for infections of bacteria, yeast, mould etc. Use it wherever eucalyptus might otherwise be indicated (*eg* respiratory conditions) and in steam baths for acne and other inflammations.

ADDITIONAL INFORMATION   When Captain Cook's expedition arrived in Australia, evidently suffering withdrawal symptoms from the cup that cheers, the crew are said to have used the fragrant leaves of *melaleuca* species as a substitute – hence the name tea tree.

The oil is a relative newcomer to aromatherapy but has already earned itself a reputation especially with regard to its antiseptic and (supposed) anti-viral action. Tea tree is closely related to cajaput and niaouli but neither of these compares in terms of antiseptic value.

An interesting pamphlet *Tea Tree Oil – a medicine Kit in a bottle* was published in the 1990s. (Susan Drury – ISBN 0 8520 7 238 4). The book is disappointing in that it contains no chemical information but useful insofar as it contains brief case histories and interesting sections on particular conditions which respond well to treatment with this oil.

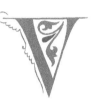

VETIVERT

NAME Vetivert

BOTANICAL NAME Vetivera Zizanoides

YIELD 2% - 3% of the dried root.

SOURCE The grass grows in India, The Philippines and China although the best oil is distilled in Europe from imported dried roots.

SPECIFIC GRAVITY At 15 degrees C vetivert oil is heavier than water – at higher temperatures it is lighter. The accuracy of given figures for specific gravity is therefore dubious but 1.015 — 1.030 (at 15 degrees C) is a good general guideline.

MAJOR CHEMICAL CONSTITUENTS vetivenol, vetivene.

METHOD OF EXTRACTION By steam distillation of the ground up roots digested in water.

COLOUR Dark brown, sometimes with a greenish tinge. Vetivert oils from some sources cause ethanol to turn green.

SAFETY DATA Safe within the usual guidelines.

PERFUMERY USES In fine perfumes as a fixative – traces for floral types – greater quantities for heavy, oriental types.

ADDITIONAL INFORMATION The Vedas advise the spiritual man to build his house near kusha (vetivert) grass so that his meditations might be enhanced by the fragrance. Fans made from the grass occasionally appear on the European market. The *Pharmacopia Indica* mentions the discovery of two copper plates dating from the twelfth century which mention vetivert among items subject to taxation. The actual term used is *turushkadanda* meaning aromatic grass or reed.

YLANG YLANG

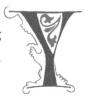

NAME Ylang Ylang, alan guilan, ihlang ihlang, all meaning 'flower of flowers' or 'perfume of perfumes' depending on who you believe.

BOTANICAL NAME Cananga Odorata

YIELD 1 – 2%. More for inferior distillations.

SOURCE Reunion, Philippines, Java, Sumatra.

SPECIFIC GRAVITY 0.930 – 0.950

COLOUR yellow to dark yellow

MAJOR CHEMICAL CONSTITUENTS para-cresyl-methyl ether, geraniol, linalool, cadinene, pinene, benzyl alcohol, iso-eugenol, methyl salicylate, benzyl benzoate, safrol, valeric acid.

METHOD OF EXTRACTION Steam distillation of the flowers.

SAFETY DATA Safe within the usual guidelines but some therapists prefer to use greater dilutions than 3% in order to avoid headaches – theirs, not the clients.

THERAPEUTIC USES Ylang ylang finds much application in the treatment of conditions resulting from stress, anxiety and misemotion and is claimed to be aphrodisiac, presumably because of its calming properties and its direct effect on the sympathetic nervous system as identified by Professor Torii of Toho University in Japan. It is a good tonic for both dry and oily skin.

PERFUMERY USES Reminiscent of hyacinth, ylang ylang is a heady, floral perfume but is much cheaper than other oils in the same category. It is used in quality perfumes, its cheaper counterpart, *cananga oil*, replacing it in inexpensive and soap perfumes. Artificial violet and lilac perfumes often include ylang ylang as a modifier. Much used in 'heavy, oriental' types of perfume.

ATTRIBUTION Maybe Venus.

ADDITIONAL INFORMATION Ylang ylang oil is extracted from the yellow (*ie* fully mature) flowers of a tall species of tree which was first identified by John Ray (1628-1705) although the oil was not produced until the 1860s and did not achieve widespread recognition until it was exhibited at the Paris Industrial Exposition of 1878.

There are several grades of ylang oil which are commercially available.

These include:- Extra, grade 1, grade 2, grade 3 and *cananga oil* which is distilled from the same species but

with less regard for quality than yield. Extra is used in fine fragrances. I recommend therapists to use grade 1 but not 2, 3 or *cananga.*

Like some of the citrus oils ylang has a tendency to become cloudy in cold conditions. It doesn't need to be filtered or thrown away. Just put it somewhere a little warmer and wait for the waxes to go back into solution.

If you have an interest in aromatherapy and you believe, as I do, that the use of essential oils as medicines should be taken more seriously, please report any companies making therapeutic claims in print to the MHRA*. Write your complaint to

MHRA, Borderline Section, 16th Floor, Market Towers, 19 Elms Lane, London SW8 5NQ.

The MHRA is obliged to follow up every complaint.

Medicines and Healthcare Products Regulatory Agency.

12

Therapeutic Index

with occasional comments

The following index is a guideline only. It should not be taken to be prescriptive. Your appraisal of your patient and your intuition as to which materials might be most appropriate to use are of the greatest importance. Use an index such as this one if you're stuck and don't know which way to go. This index is not intended to be exhaustive and I've commented only where I have a particular point to make or an interesting anecdote to offer.

ABRASIONS patchouli, lavender, chamomile

ABSCESS lavender, garlic[1]

ACNE tea tree, lavender[2]

ALOPECIA lavender, palma rosa, rosemary

ANTISEPTICS virtually all essential oils may be considered antiseptic

APPETITE (LOSS OF) lemongrass, vanilla, fennel, ginger

ARTHRITIS evening primrose oil, frankincense, eucalyptus, rosemary, cypress

ASTHMA frankincense, lavender, peppermint(mentha piperita), pine, benzoin, ravensara

BRITTLE NAILS lemon

BRONCHITIS frankincense, benzoin, pine, eucalyptus, ravensara, lavender

BURNS lavender

CATARRH peppermint(mentha arvensis), eucalyptus

CELLULITIS juniperberry, lavender, wheatgerm

CHICKEN-POX geranium[3]

CHILLBLAINS lemon, copaiba

COLDS eucalyptus, lemon, ravensara

CONSTIPATION fennel, black pepper, ginger

CONTAGION tea tree, orange, clovebud, cinnamon, lavender

COUGH benzoin, eucalyptus, ravensara, lavender[4]

CUTS patchouli, lavender

DEBILITY (GENERAL) bergamot, mandarin

DERMATITIS lavender, chamomile Roman, chamomile German

DEPRESSION patchouli, mandarin, valerian, rose absolute, petitgrain

DISINFECTION (OF ENVIRONMENTS) orange, tea tree, thyme, lavender

DYSPEPSIA peppermint (piperita), fennel

EARACHE niaouli, cajaput

ECZEMA (SKIN BROKEN AND BLEEDING) patchouli

ECZEMA (DRY) lavender, geranium, rose otto, wheatgerm, sweet almond

ECZEMA (WEEPING) lavender, juniperberry

EMPHYSEMA frankincense, eucalyptus, camphor

EPILEPSY rosemary in minute doses

FEET (ATHLETE'S FOOT) peppermint (piperita), lavender[5]

FEET (SMELLY) peppermint (piperita), lavender

FEVER eucalyptus, lemon

FLATULENCE fennel, ginger, peppermint (piperita)

GENITO URINARY INFECTIONS sandalwood, juniperberry

GINGIVITIS myrrh, lemon, clove-bud [6]

GONORRHOEA lavender, sandalwood

GOUT geranium, juniperberry, rosemary

GRIEF rose absolute, mandarin, bergamot, lime

HAIRCARE grapefruit, rosemary, lavender

HEADACHE lavender, patchouli

HERPES (COLD SORE) geranium[7]

IMPETIGO chamomile[8]

IMPOTENCE patchouli, clary sage, jasmin, ylang, aloewood

INFLUENZA tea tree, manuka

INFLUENZA (SIDE-INFECTION BY BACTERIA) tea tree, lavender, peppermint (any)

INSECT BITES lavender

INSECTS (TO REPEL) citronella, lemongrass, sandalwood, cedarwood

INSOMNIA lavender, patchouli, hop, valerian

LARYNGITIS sandalwood, cajaput, eucalyptus, ravensara[9]

LEUCORRHOEA lavender

LICE tea tree, lavender, lemon, orange terpenes, rosemary[10]

MEMORY (POOR) basil

MENSTRUATION (PAINFUL) clary sage, peppermint (piperita)

MEASLES ravensara

MIGRAINE lavender

ORAL HYGIENE tea tree, thyme, eucalyptus

PALPITATIONS neroli, peppermint (piperita), rosemary
PILES myrrh, lavender
PNEUMONIA eucalyptus, frankincense, ravensara, pine
PSORIASIS coconut oil[11]

RHEUMATOID ARTHRITIS evening primrose, frankincense, eucalyptus, rosemary, cypress

SEXUAL DEBILITY ylang, aloewood, damiana, davana
SHINGLES geranium [3]
SINUSITIS eucalyptus, ravensara, peppermint (arvensis)
SKINCARE cedarwood, grapefruit
SUNBURN lavender, coconut oil

THRUSH geranium, lavender
TOOTHACHE clovebud
THROAT (SORE) sandalwood, benzoin, ginger, lemon[9]

VARICOSE VEINS myrrh, cypress

WARTS (HANDS AND FEET) lemon, (GENITAL & OTHER) sweet marjoram
WOUNDS patchouli, lavender, yarrow
WOUNDS (INFECTED) patchouli, lavender, tea tree, honey
WRINKLES lemon, neroli, frankincense, rose

Notes

1. In the early weeks that Michael and I were running Id Aromatics, a woman came in to ask if I could do anything for facial abscesses. This was pretty scary stuff for me at that time (bearing in mind that we'd opened as a perfumery!) but, nevertheless, I looked through the very scant aromatherapy materials available to me at that time and concluded that lavender was the oil to use. Yes, this was even before the time that everyone used lavender for any condition that didn't have a specific oil indicated.

   The woman's concern was actually for her husband who suffered periodically from abscesses which were so bad that he was hospitalised two or three times a year. I have always been honest with people about my expertise, or more particularly, lack of it. If I don't know how to treat a condition I don't pretend that I do. In this case I said to the woman that it might be worth trying lavender oil, applied directly to the abscess as soon as it started to appear. That's really the end of the story.

   The woman continued to buy an occasional bottle of lavender oil and her husband was not hospitalised again during the nine years that I was running the shop. Treatments don't need to be complex. The simpler the better.

   At around this time someone passed an absolute to me which was sticking like toffee to a cellophane sheet. There was enough of this expensive material to make it worth my while to dissolve the absolute in alcohol and then separate the absolute out again. The first stage was easy. The second stage would have been easy had I not decided to overlook safety in the interest of speed.

What I needed to do was to remove the alcohol from the absolute. I could have done this by putting the solution on a wide shallow vessel in a sunny window. This would have taken a couple of hours. I could have set up a reflex column to vent the highly volatile fumes away from the source of heat but that would have meant going down two floors to the lab, sorting out the gear carrying it back up to the kitchen, setting it all up which would add fifty minutes to a job I could do in a saucepan if I were careful. I was careful, but not careful enough.

A momentary distraction caused me to tip the pin from horizontal ever so slightly. But that was enough for the heavy volatile vapours to cascade down the outside of the pan to the gas. Instantaneously there was a wall of fire across the kitchen from floor to ceiling. Furthermore, my hand was on fire being now covered in an oily alcohol mixture not dissimilar in its effects, I imagine, to napalm. At times like this the triage process of prioritisation kicks in. Naturally, I needed to put out the fire in the kitchen first, before it had chance to spread. That was actually quite easily done but I guess that, by this time, my hand had been on fire for about thirty seconds.

By the time I plunged it into a sink of cold water it had already been very badly burned. In fact, by the time I'd plucked up the courage to take a proper look, it was immediately apparent that the damage was severe. The thumb knuckle nearest to the hand was exposed, as were the muscle tissue and the tendons which operate the thumb. In short, my hand looked like something from a particularly unpleasant horror movie - truly nasty.

The incident, as you might expect, reminded me of of

Gattefosse. Widely regarded as the 'father' of aromatherapy, he'd used pure lavender oil into which he'd plunged his arm after a similar accident to mine. He used lavender because it was the only cold liquid available. His immediate observation was that the pain caused by such a large and serious burn was quickly soothed by the lavender oil and his later observation, when he assessed the injury some months later, was that the scarring he'd expected to be left with was nowhere near as disfiguring as he'd been expecting.

Because I had cold water available I used that immediately. Cooling the site of a burn as soon as possible after sustaining a burn of whatever severity is crucial to providing the best treatment possible. If this isn't done, the flesh will continue to cook and the injury will deteriorate further.

For about four hours after I burned my hand, I stood by the kitchen sink dipping my hand into the water and taking it out again, occasionally changing the water when it started to warm up. The reason for the in - out - in - out was to make use of Gattefosse's experience. I'd put a couple of millilitres of lavender oil into the sink. Obviously, the oil floats on water, so, to deliver it to the site of the injury, the burn has to be moved through the floating oil.

The process of treating the burn in this way was, indeed, soothing. It still hurt like hell but nowhere near as much as it had to begin with. This was the only treatment I did. I decided that recovery would take place more quickly if I didn't dress the burn. The greatest difficulty with this was that other people could see the injury and some folk almost fainted at the sight of it. I was aware that there was a danger of the wound going septic, but I was ready for that and prepared to take the risk for the benefit of a quick healing process with as little scar-tissue as possible.

Despite Gattefosse's description, I was very surprised at the final outcome. Within a couple of months, my hand was entirely back to normal. Not only were the flesh and skin fully restored, the hair follicles were back, even where the flesh and skin had been totally burned away, and, even more amazingly, the follicles were in full, hair producing, working order! In fact, the only change which had occurred was that the melanin had not been restored at the crest of the thumb-knuckle so, in summer, there's a pale patch of skin about the size of a penny.

Occasionally I get dragged in to colleges to speak to aromatherapy students. When they ask me, and they nearly always do, "What's your favourite synergistic blend?", I ask them why they want to blend such complex chemical packages as essential oils together. The reply comes back as if by rote "To balance the base, middle and top notes". This is a ridiculous proposition which comes out of having people more used to running beauty parlours than dealing with illness calling the shots when it comes to qualifications.

Balancing base, middle and top notes is a perfumers job and it is a difficult task in itself, let alone the inclusion of a healing principle. Furthermore, if you blend oils together it is more difficult to discover the active constituent. If that active constituent is the orange oil (very cheap) that you blended with rose and sandalwood (both expensive) your blend is much more expensive than it needs to be and much less ecologically sensitive. When I was working in the shop I aimed to provide remedies at about one twelfth of the current cost of a prescription.

2. An article in *The Lancet* in the early nineties concluded that tea tree oil was just as effective in the treatment of acne as benzoyl peroxide and without the unpleasant side-effects.

3. Chicken-pox and shingles respond well to geranium used in the bathwater.

4. Recent research (2005) suggests that the best remedy for cough is chocolate. More recently dark chocolate has been found to lower cholesterol (One piece per day).

5. **A Formula for the Treatment of Athlete's Foot**
    Athlete's foot is controlled very easily. I use lavender and peppermint (*mentha piperita*) in a footbath, about four drops of each. The water should be warm rather than hot. About fifteen minutes should be spent treading the water so that the toes are constantly passing through the film of oil which floats on the surface of the water.

6. A few years ago, a client who was having a mad panic phoned me. "My dentist says that if I can't get rid of this gum infection he's going to have to take all my teeth out. The tea tree's just not working." Not at all surprised about that I recommended clove bud oil to be used in water as a mouthwash. It's widely known that clove oil is a brilliant analgesic in the case of toothache. What's not widely acknowledged is that in former times, when a dentist had drilled the caries out of a tooth he would then line the

cavity with clove oil, virtually paint the hole, before putting in the amalgam. That way, if a tiny bit of infection remained, the clove would kill it, thereby avoiding further problems such as abscesses. My client used the clove for a few days and got a clean bill of health from her dentist. Clove leaf and stem oils are available but these should not be used in oral hygiene.

7. Occasionally, usually when I'm in strong sunshine for the first time in a while, a cold sore will break out on my lip. The immune system takes a dip while the body's getting used to ultra-violet light. If I catch the blister before it forms, just as the first prickles start, I apply geranium oil neat and directly. Then I forget about it because the blister doesn't form. If I catch it later the geranium works efficiently but I'm stuck with a fat lip for a couple of days (which is still much better than a week or more). Strangely, a client once reported to me that she'd successfully treated a cold sore with rose perfume. Thinking about this when I had some free time it occurred to me that geraniol, the chief component of geranium oil, is also one of the main ingredients of any rose perfume.

8. Impetigo is notoriously difficult to treat and horrifyingly contagious. Serious outbreaks have been noted in recent years among travelling communities – the folk who were referred to in the eighties as 'New Age Travellers'. The nick-name given to it by these communities – 'Septic Death' – gives an idea of its nature.

    When she was two, my daughter caught impetigo from another little girl whose sores had been diagnosed as eczema by her doctor. I have to admit that, because we were imminently about to go on a sunshine holiday, we permitted our own doctor to prescribe antibiotics, which is something we wouldn't have done at a more relaxed time.

However, having realised that this horrible condition is caused by *staphylococcus aureus* (one of the bug's that achieved super status in our ill-run hospitals) and having read what Jean Valnet has to say about this bacterium in his superb book *The Practice of Aromatherapy*, I determined to treat some of the lesions with Roman chamomile.

What Valnet says is this: "The bacteriostatic action of azulene [a fatty component of chamomile oils, RS], is produced at a concentration of 1 part in 2000 against *staphylococcus aureus, haemolytic streptococcus,* and *proteus vulgaris* in particular. Infected wounds have been healed using concentrations of from 1 part in 85,000 to 1 part in 170,000."

Accordingly I chose a few lesions and treated them exclusively with chamomile. The ones treated were the first to heal and disappear. For several years I've been telling a number of people involved in clinical trials of tea tree in respect of MRSA, the resistant form of *staph aureus,* that they're studying the effects of the wrong oil and that they should be looking at chamomiles and perhaps coconut oil, because of its high lauric acid content. To date, my words have fallen on stony ground.

9. The best treatment I ever found for sore throat is sandalwood oil. When I feel the first dryness occurring I put three or four drops of Mysore sandalwood (NOT the so-called West Indian Sandalwood) on the palm of my

hand and lick it off. Sandalwood is a much gentler oil than any of the other essential oils and is quite safe to use in this way. If you perform this treatment early enough, the sore-throat is already sorted out.

10. Infestation by head-lice is a problem which has been dramatically increasing over the past few years, I suspect as a result of warmer winters, fitted carpets, central heating and double-glazing. The kinds of hermetically sealed environments which we typically occupy these days must have greatly improved the life-style of the louse. If you ask your pharmacist, the chances are you'll be supplied with an organo-phosphate, the same stuff that's used in sheep-dip and which causes all manner of health hazards for farmers who are stupid enough to use it.

That's the last thing you want to put on you or your child's head. Tea tree gets rid of critters in the hair as does rosemary. If I ever encounter the problem myself, my money's on orange terpenes, chemicals which have been removed from orange oil and which are, in themselves, considerably safer than orange oil itself for this kind of purpose.

Orange terpenes could also be used to clean up oils spills on the shoreline. The terpenes bind to the oil and form a hard substance which sinks to the bottom and causes no further problem. This natural solution to a massive environmental problem has never been taken up because orange terpenes cost a few pence more per litre than the less efficient chemicals which the market prefers to use.

11. Psoriasis presents its own problems. It can't be treated

like eczema or dermatitis and its roots are nearly always in personal trauma. My own instinct is to treat the trauma (patchouli, frankincense, counseling etc.) rather than the skin, but there is a topical lotion which helps.

The skin can become uncomfortably scaly, itchy and unsightly. Apply coconut oil, a tiny amount is enough, to moisturise the affected areas. This softens the scales and relieves some of the discomfort at the same time as rendering the scales more transparent. If the face, hands and forearms are affected this is very important since an individual's self-esteem can be, at least partially restored, if his appearance is deemed more acceptable.

Other skin conditions tend to respond favourably to vitamin E. Psoriasis does not. *In extremis* psoriasis speeds up the formation and development of skin cells so that as little as twelve days might complete the cycle and the skin cell is sloughed off. Vitamin E encourages the development of skin cells while, what is most needed in psoriasis is to slow that process down.

13

Miscellaneous Information
Frequently Asked Questions

HOW DO I KNOW IF AN ESSENTIAL OIL IS PURE?
Essential oils are, by definition, pure. A better question to ask is:

ARE THE ESSENTIAL OILS AVAILABLE OF GOOD QUALITY? Apologies for putting it like that but any or all of the kitchen sink aromatherapy operations which have proliferated over the past few years can offer 'pure' essential oils – there's no difficulty involved in that. Of much greater importance is whether the oil is a) of good enough quality to use therapeutically and b) the right chemotype to use therapeutically.

For example, you might find a half-price sandalwood – it would be pure – it would also be useless. You can't appraise sandalwood just by sniffing the bottle or even by tasting. You need a first distillation, not an oil produced from wood that's already been 'squeezed out'. If you use the wrong chemotype of an oil you probably won't get the result you're looking for and in some cases, basil for example, you run the risk of using a toxic substance on your client. (See info on basil in Monographs).

WHAT DOSAGES SHOULD I USE?

I can't give information that will suit all cases all the time and if you're in any doubt at all DON'T DO IT. However, it is sensible to say that essential oils are so powerful that our senses are unable to convey that power. Using less of an essential oil is virtually always better than using more.

IN MASSAGE SOLUTIONS
about 3% essential oil to 97% fixed oil
IN THE BATHWATER four drops
IN A FOOTBATH four drops

Many books suggest larger dosages than this. Please ignore them. The author of a book can tell you anything. I've been constrained by law for the past twenty-five years (while I was selling essential oils) and consequently I'm very comfortable with being careful.

WHAT'S THE DIFFERENCE BETWEEN
LAVENDER BP & LAVENDER

40/42%? BP (British Pharmacopeia) is an old fashioned attempt to standardize botanical drugs. As far as lavender is concerned the BP requires the oil to contain a minimum of 39% of esters, most important of these being linalyl acetate. 40/42 is a more international standard, introduced more recently, and which requires the oil to contain, you guessed it, between 40 and 42 percent of the same constituent. The linalyl acetate content has little effect on the odour of the oil, this being more to do with ethyl amyl ketone.

WHAT DOES IT MEAN WHEN AN OIL IS SAID TO BE BERGAPTEN FREE?

This specifically refers to bergamot oil which contains, amongst many other constituents, a group of furocoumarins, one of which, *bergapten,* is known to sensitize the skin in the presence of UV light. In some individuals this can cause permanent patchy brown pigmentation to occur. This sensitization can be avoided by staying out of the sun after a treatment with bergamot or by using a rectified bergamot from which the furocoumarins have been removed. For the same reason some suppliers offer distilled lime and lemon. The process of distillation provides a safer oil to use than the more common, pressed fruit oils.

DO I NEED TO ADD SOMETHING TO ESSENTIAL OIL BEFORE I PUT IT IN THE BATH-WATER?

Some people like to use an emulsifier such as cows' milk, fixed oil, or sulphated castor oil – a marvelous idea if you don't mind spending half an hour cleaning the bath afterwards! Apart from pure hedonism there are two practical reasons for using essential oil in the bath-water. One is that the warm water encourages the evaporation of the oil so that elements of it are inhaled. The second is that four drops of oil will spread to form a film over the entire surface of the water. Warm water makes the skin more receptive to all oils of vegetable origin. This means that when the body comes out of the water, pre-prepared by warming, it moves through the film of oil and receives a very thin film of oil of its own. Because the skin is extra absorbent as far as oil is concerned, the oil is quickly picked up by the blood stream and, to a lesser extent by the lymphatic fluid. The lavender, or whatever, is found in traces in the major organs within half an hour or so.

ESSENTIAL OILS ARE NATURAL AND THEREFORE SAFE PRODUCTS AREN'T THEY?

Essential oils are produced by nature but it's a bit of a stretch to say that they are natural. Yes, you can pop the oil out of orange rind by poking a thumbnail into it. Do this near a candle-flame and you'll see the tiny drops of oil combusting – entirely natural. If you collected the oil from half a ton of orange rind, would the product still be natural? In any case most essential oils have to be teased out of the plant parts by distillation and in a lot of cases, chamomile for example, chemicals not present in the plant show up in the oil as a by-product of the process. In the case of chamomile, azulene, possibly the most useful element in this essential oil, arises as a by-product.

It's very difficult to assess the strength of an essential oil because we're simply not equipped to appraise anything so strong. Try diluting an oil 100 times and see if you can smell it next day. If your nose works at all, you'll smell it.

Treat essential oils with respect. They are extremely complex chemical packages and their natural origin, although this qualifies them as better medicines than their pharmaceutical counterparts, does not mean that they can be used indefinitely or recklessly. Always check out specific safety data before using an oil. Check for contra-indications. Patch test before massaging. All the above refers to 3% dilutions, not just to neat oil!

14

What's going on with Tea Tree Oil?

This commodity is available in two grades, pharmaceutical and cosmetic. The grade is dependant on whether the oil is high or low in terpinen 4ol. However, because the pharmaceutical grade commands a much higher price than the cosmetic grade, it seems to have become standard practice amongst many Australian growers/distillers to keep back batches which are terpinen 4ol poor and to blend this with batches which are terpinen 4ol rich, thereby satisfying the criteria for pharmaceutical grade oil for all or most of the oil they produce.*

---

*There is a widespread belief that gas chromatography reveals everything that one might want to know about the chemistry of an oil. While this is true to a limited extent GCs cannot reveal whether or not an oil has been blended.

As far as I'm concerned an essential oil comes, by definition, from a single source and should not be a blended material.

For the above reason I now obtain tea tree oil from a plantation in Bungawalbyn where, I am assured, this spurious blending does not take place. In addition to this, sheep are grazed in the tea tree paddocks and this provides a virtually organic product. Look for *Bungawalbyn* on the label. This is the epicentre of quality tea tree oil production.

The year 1999-2000 saw the demise of many small plantations in Australia, especially those whose oil output was not of the highest quality. In order to cushion bankruptcies, much of this poor quality oil has been dumped into the UK market. Most of it is not at all suitable for medical use but there is no way the end user can tell just by smelling it whether or not an oil is terpinen 4ol rich. The ancient advice to buy from a supplier you know applies more now than it ever did before.

EXAMPLE MATERIAL DATA SHEET –
Tea tree oil (Bungawalbyn) Batch H6932

MAJOR CONSTITUENTS
terpinen 4 ol (40.82%), 1,8 cineole, limonene, alpha pinene, para cymene, alpha terpinene, terpinolene, gamma terpinene, alpha terpineol, sabinene, aromadendrene, viridiflourine, delta cadinene, globulol, viridiflourol.
SPECIFIC GRAVITY @ 20 DEG C O.893
REFRACTIVE INDEX " " "   1.4806
OPTICAL ROTATION " " '   +9.7 deg
SOLUBILITY IN 85% ETHANOL (V/V) AT 20 deg C 0.6

15

A Further Note On Health & Safety

There recently emerged a suggestion that blending safe essential oils together might result in the compounding of hazardous chemicals not present in the individual oils themselves. This does not occur with oils which have GRAS status; that is, oils which, internationally, are Generally Recognized As Safe. This group typically includes all the oils which are currently used in aromatherapy and other disciplines of natural medicine.

The opposite end of the spectrum of essential oil safety data is occupied by very few oils which are, in any case, never offered to therapists or to the general public. Most hazardous among these is mustard oil which is used in the production of mustard gas. Other oils which should not be used by therapists are listed in *OILS WHICH SHOULD NOT BE USED IN*

AROMATHERAPY (q.v.).

Aromatherapists blend oils in order to create synergies where the action of certain components of one oil is supported by the action of components of another. Having created a synergy, though, the therapist will then dilute the mixture to less than 3% in a bland oil such as fractionated coconut.

Clients should be patch tested routinely in aromatherapy each time a new oil or synergy is used. Patch-testing is a standard procedure which ensures that a full body massage is not given to a client who might be irritated by a particular oil or blend. In practice, 99.99% of patch tests are negative but they serve to reassure (principally) the therapist that no untoward reactions are likely to occur following a treatment.

16

Oils which should not be used in aromatherapy

There are thousands of essential oils, produced for uses as diverse as flavourings for liqueurs to perfumes for boot polish. Many of the oils offered for sale and, indeed, a good number of oils referred to in aromatherapy books, should not be used at all by therapists, mostly because they are toxic at the level of dilution used in aromatherapy (typically about 3%).

Suppliers these days tend to be careful about which oils they offer. Most have GRAS status – that is, they are Generally Recognized As Safe.

The following is a list of oils which, for whatever reason, should **not** be used in aromatherapy at all under any circumstances:-

Inula helenium, jaborandi leaf, lavender cotton,

southernwood, basil (exotic), pennyroyal, thuja, wintergreen, wormwood, rue, clove-stem, (clove-leaf and clove-bud should be used on the skin with extreme caution), **pimento leaf,** *buchu, opoponax, peru balsam, ajowan, wormseed, tansy, sassafras, mustard, mugwort, horseradish, costus, cinnamon bark, cassia, calamus, boldo leaf, bitter almond.*

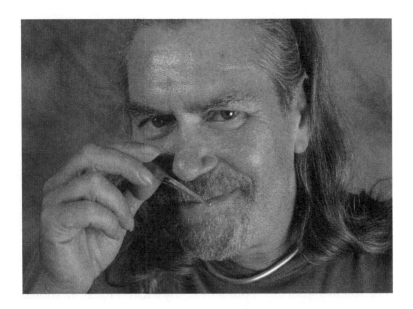

Ray 2005, snapped at a photo shoot where he was helping out. Photo by Nigel Mullaney of Phoenix Creative Media with whom Ray made the Album 'The end of the world' in 1997.

17

Health & Safety Data regarding the Storage & Handling of Essential Oils (COSHH)

The observations in these notes are particularly applicable to the handling of industrial quantities of essential oils. The potential health & safety problems outlined below are hardly likely to arise in the therapeutic situation typically using 10ml amounts of essential oils. Nevertheless, all individuals using essential oils should be aware of standard procedures in the unlikely event of mishap. See also 'Using aromatherapy products at home'.

Essential oils are highly complex mixtures of organic chemicals principally made up of alcohols, esters, ketones and phenols. In their undiluted state they should not be applied to the skin or ingested. Storage in a dark place at room temperature is advised.

Most of the oils currently offered have GRAS status – that is, they are Generally Recognized As Safe.

GENERAL Keep essential oils away from foodstuffs and out of reach of children and animals. Follow good housekeeping procedures.

FIRE Work in a well ventilated area away from sources of ignition. Wipe up spills immediately and dispose of wipes in a fire-safe bin. All essential oils are volatile and become potentially hazardous when they are absorbed into organic materials such as sawdust or paper. In industrial situations CO_2, foam or dry powder extinguishers are applicable. Do not use water.

HEALTH AND SAFETY

INGESTION In the unlikely event, do not induce vomitting. Seek medical attention. Contact your supplier quoting the product name and the batch number. If there is no batch number, don't buy from that source again. It is illegal in the UK to supply oils without batch numbers.

INHALATION In the very unlikely event, seek medical attention and contact your supplier.

EYE CONTACT Irrigate copiously with cold (preferably sterile) water. If stinging persists after ten minutes, seek medical attention and contact your supplier.

18

A Quick Note On: Benzoin, Peru, Galbanum, Immortelle, Oak-Moss, Aniseed, Jojoba, Sandalwood, Fragrance & Rose Otto.

At first glance it might seem that there is little to connect the items listed above, but of all the aromatic products widely in use these commodities are occasionally rather difficult to handle. Benzoin, galbanum, immortelle and oakmoss, because they are resinoids or absolutes which behave like resinoids, tend towards being semi-solid when they are cold. Most suppliers dilute these materials in order to make them pourable. As far as I'm concerned, dilution defeats the object when all that's required is the application of warmth. If you experience handling difficulties with these resinoids, remove the bottle cap and dropper and stand the bottle on a central-heating radiator or similar. This kind of treatment does not denature the material and it is standard treatment in professional perfume houses to keep resinoids in special warm cupboards.

While you may experience similar difficulties with aniseed and jojoba this is for quite different reasons. Aniseed freezes at 55f and will become liquid again if you keep it in a pocket for a few minutes. Jojoba sets solid when it is cool because it is, itself, a wax and not an oil. Here again a pocket should warm it enough to render it liquid.

Rose otto is a different matter again. Most rose ottos remain liquid at all reasonable temperatures. However, the very best quality Bulgarian rose otto (the kind that I use) congeals at low temperatures. You don't need to warm this to liquify it – just shake it vigorously for a few seconds.

19

Fixed Oils (also known as carrier oils, vegetable oils)

Fixed oils are, by definition, non-volatile, and are used in aromatherapy to perform two functions:-

1. To dilute essential oils and blends of essential oils to an appropriate strength.
2. To 'carry' the essential oils through the skin and into the bloodstream and lymph system.

FRACTIONATED COCONUT OIL There are many fixed oils available - apricot kernel, avocado, olive, groundnut (arachis), grapeseed, etc. I use fractionated coconut oil for 99% of treatments. Coconut is a fine, odourless oil, readily absorbed by the skin. It also has the advantage of being stable. The other fixed oils (mentioned above) can go rancid or ropey fairly quickly and some can start to form sediments almost immediately.

For massage preparations use 97% fractionated coconut to 3% essential oils unless otherwise indicated by safety data.

STRETCH MARKS Pure fractionated coconut oil with no

additives is useful in the treatment of stretch marks. The oil should be daily massaged into the affected area(s) using a gentle pinching action. It is best to start this treatment as soon as the marks begin to appear (often during pregnancy). Treating stretch marks when the damage has already been done is a more difficult, but not insurmountable, problem.

DRY, SENSITIVE SKIN For dry or sensitive skin fractionated coconut oil may be added to the bathwater. Add a few drops of essential oil to 500ml of FCO. To avoid the problem of the oil sticking to the bath rather than the body add two tablespoons of mild shampoo to the mixture.

MATURE SKIN Add ten drops of FCO to 30ml of soya yoghurt. Cream these together and add two drops of lavender oil. Apply a thin film of the product to the face and leave it for five minutes. Rinse off with cold water.

DRY, DULL HAIR Wet the hair slightly and massage in FCO which has been warmed by placing the bottle in hot water. Use a hot, wet towel as a turban and leave it on for as long as possible, preferably overnight. Wash out with shampoo.

WHEATGERM OIL This is another fixed oil worthy of mention. Too viscous to be used as a carrier oil it is very rich in tocopherols and consequently useful in the treatment of wounds, abrasions, cuts and skin conditions such as eczema and dermatitis. Tocopherols stimulate the production of skin cells and help the skin to heal more quickly. [NB Do not use wheatgerm oil to treat psoriasis since one of the problems here is that skin cells are formed and sloughed off much more quickly than they are by normal skin]. 2% - 3% of wheatgerm added to a massage oil helps retard the oxidisation process and increases shelf-life. If you use fractionated coconut oil you do not need to be concerned about this.

20

How to Copy A Perfume

Commercial perfumes are not easy for the home enthusiast to copy. The professional perfumer has many hundreds of aromatic substances from which to choose, most of which are not available to the amateur. In addition to essential oils and absolutes he will have pure synthetics which need to be handled very carefully. I once accidentally transferred an invisible amount of para-cresyl acetate on to my hand. Naturally, I attempted to wash it off immediately. When soap and water failed, having actually made the smell stronger, I resorted to 99% alcohol which had the same effect. Over the next day or two the smell got stronger and stronger and wherever I went I exuded the overpowering smell of May-blossom.

The perfumer also has aldehydes and other powerful odour

chemicals as well as exalters, chemicals which have the effect of 'lifting' a finished perfume.

Whether you're trying to copy a complex commercial perfume or a straightforward blend of oils, the method is the same. Imagine that your sense of smell works like one of those simple cognitive tests often imposed on children where wooden shapes fit perfectly into wooden holes if the correct hole has been selected. Once the hole is filled, obviously nothing else can go in there.

The sense of smell functions like that. If you overpower it with one smell, there comes a point where you can't detect that smell any more.

So - have a quick sniff of the perfume you'd like to copy, preferably on a smelling paper so that you're not going to pick up any stray smells from your hands or elsewhere. What's the first impression? Let's say there's a strong ylang note. Get your bottle of ylang and smell it very deliberately until you've 'keyed it out'. Then smell your sample again. It's slightly simpler this time because the ylang's not getting in the way. What's the next impression? Repeat the process and keep going until you can't smell anything at all.

You need to take long breaks in fresh air. Sometimes it's good to leave a smelling strip overnight. This gives the volatile components time to escape completely, leaving only base notes behind. Treat the base notes as before in order to simplify their identification.

21

Two Poems

Since this is the nearest I'm likely to get to autobiography, I include two poems here. Both have been published several times already, and they have little to do with aromatics and more to do with memoir.

The first, *The Book of the Apple I want to Eat*, I wrote in Cairo in 1981. The second, *The Singing Tadpole*, I wrote in Morton in 1987.

I published it myself in pamphlet form with an accompanying sound cassette which I recorded at Black Edge Farm Studio in one take. I then added music using synthesizers and a stringed instrument I made for the purpose.

Because of its 'Celtic Twilight' associations, it received a special commendation from the W B Yeats Society in Oxford. This is, in my view, my best work.

The Singing Tadpole

or

The Pig in the Pond

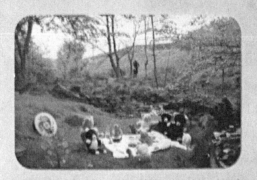

(an invitation from chaos)

by

THESSALONIUS LOYOLA

The Singing Tadpole. When I issued the poem in 1987 it was as a sound poem on cassette. Fifty copies of the cassette were issued with a booklet which contained the text of the poem and notes explaining the more difficult passages.

The Book of the Apple I want to Eat

I am my own circle.

The irreconcilabilities of dream and reality may be the error of reality.

My life is not a metronome.

I am that I am is not enough. I am also the effect of things and qualities which I am not and I am as much my faults as my qualities.

I am flying solo. There is no God where I am because I do not permit him to exist; yet his absence is also a part of me and it is his absence which urges me to fly.

The Goddess is an empty dress, a quality without a form; fill the space and that space is the self confined.

Infinity is bounded by its own name.

I cast doubt into the still and stagnant for the ripple of change that's in it.

The All is unchanging but the ripples reach its rim, repercussive, and return to 'suage the axletree.

At the centre is stability. The hub is the heart that pounds the power of love, the yoke of speed and stillness, spinning the balance of speed and inertia.

I maintain my place, a dervish disciple caught on the coals - dancing!

I taught myself to dance; my body to be still.

Lie with me now for when the dance begins again I shall forget.

Sweet oblivion. Every way I win.

All guests are welcome once.

Tear down these symbols wrought of memory, turning over old leaves to nourish new roots.

Today's ideas illuminate the shadows of yesterday's intentions.

No matter, the dance is spiral and the music goes on.
Listen to the rhythm of the retrograde drum.

I am offered water but shall I drink or swim? Better to swim.
Think of the homeless fish.
There is a fish that flies, to other fish a God. He knows the in and the out.
  To the bird he is a meal. Beware the God-eater.
I want out - to see in. Out there is the apple I want to eat.

I am my own pyramid, of Earth or Fire is no consequence.
I crawl the Mysteries within hoping for a secret door, but robbers were here before me and the treasures are scattered.
I become a collector.

There is no God here, but the perfume of the Goddess lingers.
When I dream tonight what colour should I choose?
The blue of water, the purple of ecstacy? The green of growing?
The green is best, for the root is stronger than the stem, drinking deep, the frond more ecstatic than the wand, dancing in the Air.

People call me black yet I absorb no light, using no more than my share.
I steal only her fragrance and that remains forever. Her perfume is on my pillow.
All but the likeness disappears for I am not the magician but the magick, and even the likeness is a part of me.

Only dead things have no seed. Only dead things have no self.

Therefore is the love of the seed and the love of the self the love of all life.

Can I kill myself for love?

There is no profit in this. Nor is any loss. The only prize the apple-seed.

Ring the changes to bring down these walls or for the joy of change.

Create and destroy are brothers. It is I who make them fight.

Posture before the mirror looking in.

There am I, looking out. Somewhere in there is the apple I want to eat.

I am my own man. The *you* and the *I* differ only in function. Function is forgery, forgery theft. We steal our masks one from the other. No matter -they are all the same. Memory is impaired by life - life by memory. To forget is to live, but to remember is to reach for the apple.

The beating of a distant drum - a drunken madness for all who hear.

With the beating of my unfledged wings I cover her call, but dare I fly?

And if I fall? Air is strong.

Naked, unmasked, I dance to the music of time, unfettered of need. I need only the apple, and that is within my grasp.

The Singing Tadpole
or
The Pig in the Pond
(an invitation from Chaos)

Three Blinks of an Eye

In the misty distance, beneath a hazeltree, a salmon leaps, splashing. Later, ungently persuaded by the force called G, he returns to his element. The two instants dis-exist, later to reform as the subtle image blocks of tainted history (if I write or remember them). But the new, fresh instant contains the salmon's leap and fall. All the fishy leaping and falling that ever was is encapsuled in its past. The potential future of this new instant, attenuated by knowledge of the salmon's leap, twists and shifts the multiversal destination. All change.

The Coracle

I sit still in my roundboat, breathless and wide-eyed, alert to the vibrant particules of happenstance exploding silently around me in the dark, unmoving air. Snake-eyed, with hunter's intent, I stalk the avenues of improbability, motionless and empty headed.

There is no star or chart to guide my way between the moments. No-one was here before.

In time long passed I teased the multiverse to tell me truth, and this I learned. That time is mine, to run it fast or slow as I choose.

In my wizardry I run time slow, finding space between the moments to sift and strain the deposits of time with pan-like perception, searching, ibis-beaked, for that instant of all instants where and when my intent is least improbable.

Then the oar goes in, my coracular craft taking direction from me, un-needful of rudder (while I know my desire). I see the salient salmon leap, but that is of no moment. I prowl a different prey, long distant, but nearer now the multiverse has changed, once again, in my favour.
If you go down to the woods tonight...

Eating my onion I deny attention to small, glittering objects in the undergrowth. I scry the canopy of leaves against the dark sky, unmindful of giant birds and looming Gods who press their images on me.

No need for eyes in this lumined dark, for feet and hands, guided by the feeling tendrils of the wyrdweb, find their own way out and home - no danger in the dark.

My onion links a taste from time before of sweet-mouthed kisses, unintended to offend, and times of magick past in this place process before the inner eye, softly forging link on link the chain that never hammer saw.

On the bank a host of figures, robed and masked, unmoving,

fix their gaze on the man with the onion, pondering his own state.

Moving again, a tree takes me, an insect in a brittle hand. I struggle to escape with slow, unfrantic movements, then give myself in calm surrender like a true - onion eater.

My surrender makes me free and I expand to fill the world between the worlds, the tree an incidental snare in a wood full of diamonds.

I join the host and all the masks are changed. It makes no difference. The Goddess, a forger herself and wise to wizardcraft, knows we are not fooled.

Bottle returned to Sender

Omar, of the old times, tried many a wise man's door, but later lamented the time mis-spent, having found his genius - in a bottle.

Following in his sagely steps I mounted an expedition to the East. The bottle I found was empty, so I breathed my own spirit in and corked it tight forever.

A bottle is always a comfort on a cold night. Some cold is caused by scrutiny. If I stare too long and hard, the magick dissolves to nothing, like a word nine times repeated or a prayer too often uttered.

The indiscriminate word tumbles from the mouth of every

would-be mage, (with or without the counterfeit courage of the bottle), regardless of time, place or meaning.

He who has ears to hear, let him listen to that reckless rhetoric - and then make up his own mind. Listen, you torturers of innocent words. I will follow you - if you will follow me.

A Feast is as good as Enough

I know a pool where the salient salmon grows fat on nuts and knowledge. I divine the instant of his capture, but should I cast a hierophantic hook or spin the web between the moments of his leap and fall?

I weave the web, avoiding hurt, and in the third instant he is mine. Glad and rejoicing that I have not caught a man as Christian folk are wont to do, I haul him in and off with his head. This I save to talk with at my leisure. The rest I spit upon an oaken hearth, moist mouthed and moody minded.

"Why did you kill me, you bastard?"

"Shut your mouth, fish-face."

"Why will you eat my body?"

"It's a sacrament. Be quiet or I'll give you to the cat." I touch the skewered salmon, testing for readiness, and burn my thumb on the sizzling skin. Hand to mouth the thumb goes in, a childish pose for the man who knows the secret of the salmon. But what he knew, now I know too. This sacrament will have a hazelnut in every bite.

Tertiary Chaos

Stars fade. Dreamy night, displaced by dawn, is slowly drawn around the world and weavers of words must wake into wide and worn industrious day. But stay! I have a point to press before lucidity is marred by cruel day. Surely we have not come thus far - to know the how and why and when - to be confounded by the what!

Not since the days of Merlin did our land abound in wizardry, as is the case today. "But", you interject, "wizardry was easy in those days. The hollow hills and henges a simple matter of material relocation. See our soaring cities!" I see our soaring cities, and from my weeping springs a stream in which the salient salmon swims sulkily to sea.

He cannot go the old-time way - our soaring city turned his river red and un-productive, a feculent fosse stinking its way to the reluctant source of life. I stalked him fair, but that was the last and final time. For when you tread that path beside the pool in time to come, you'll find no thrill in wrangling out a phosphorescent fish.

The magick works, moment by moment grows stronger. But Earth grows weak and cannot wait on prating politics. The tolerant trees whisper through the wyrd for quiet magick's aid and I choose THIS instant to plant the seed of my desire, sigil-like, in your confused imagination.

The silent power of witch and wizard, magicians diverse of cloak and creed joined just in this. To chart the Earth a different course for us to play our magick in.

BIBLIOGRAPHY

Perfume by Patrick Suskind, Pocket Books, 1986, ISBN 0-671-72595-5 (Also a fabulous film, 2007, distributed by Pathe).

Jitterbug Perfume by Tom Robbins, Bantam Books, 1996, ISBN 0-553-40383-4

The Qabalah of Aleister Crowley, (including Liber 777), Samuel Weiser, 1973, ISBN 0-87728-222-6

Frankincense and Myrrh by Nigel Groom, Longman, 1981, ISBN 0-582-76476-9

Soaps, Perfumes and Cosmetics by William A Poucher, Chapman & Hall, 1925

The Practice of Aromatherapy by Jean Valnet (trans Robert Tisserand), C W Daniel, 1988, ISBN 0-85207-143-4

The Volatile Oils by Gildemeister & Hoffman, Germania Publishing, 1899

The Book of Pleasure by Austin Osman Spare, Morton Press, 93 Publishing

Parry's Cyclopaedia of Perfumery by Ernest J Parry, Churchill, 1925

Scents and Sensuality by Max Lake, John Murray, 1989, ISBN0-7195-4600-1

Index

Mandrake
'Books you don't see everyday'

The Apophenion: A Chaos Magic Paradigm by **Peter J Carroll**

978-1869928-421, £10.99

My final Magnum Opus if its ideas remain unfalsified within my lifetime, otherwise its back to the drawing board. Yet I've tried to keep it as short and simple as possible, it consists of eight fairly brief and terse chapters and five appendices.

It attacks most of the great questions of being, free will, consciousness, meaning, the nature of mind, and humanity's place in the cosmos, from a magical perspective. Some of the conclusions seem to challenge many of the deeply held assumptions that our culture has taught us, so brace yourself for the paradigm crash and look for the jewels revealed in the wreckage.

This book contains something to offend everyone; enough science to upset the magicians, enough magic to upset the scientists, and enough blasphemy to upset most trancendentalists.

The most original, and probably the most important, writer on Magick since Aleister Crowley.

> -Robert Anton Wilson, author of the *Cosmic Trigger* trilogy.

Bright From the Well by **Dave Lee**

978-1869928-841, £10.99

'Bright From the Well' consists of five stories plus five essays and a rune-poem. The stories revolve around themes from Norse myth - the marriage of Frey and Gerd, the story of how Gullveig-Heidh reveals her powers to the gods, a modern take on the social-origins myth Rig's Tale, Loki attending a pagan pub moot and the Ragnarok seen through the eyes of an ancient shaman.

The essays include examination of the Norse creation or origins story, of the magician in or against the world and a chaoist's magical experiences looked at from the standpoint of Northern magic.'

'Dave Lee coaches breathwork, writes fiction and non-fiction, blends incenses and oils, creates music and collages'

Magick Works: cutting edge essays from the path of Pleasure, Freedom and Power by Julian Vayne

978-1869928-469 £10.99

Enter the world of the occultist: where the spirits of the dead dwell amongst us, where the politics of ecstasy are played out, and where magick spills into every aspect of life.

It's all right here; sex, drugs, witchcraft and gardening. From academic papers, through to first person accounts of high-octaine rituals. In Magick Works you will find cutting edge essays from the path of Pleasure, Freedom and Power.

In this seminal collection Julian Vayne explores;

* The Tantric use of Ketamine.
* Social Justice, Green Politics and Druidry.
* English Witchcraft and Macumba
* The Magickal use of Space.
* Cognitive Liberty and the Occult.
* Psychogeography & Chaos Magick.
* Tai Chi and Apocalyptic Paranoia.
* Self-identity, Extropianism and the Abyss.
* Parenthood as Spiritual Practice.
* Aleister Crowley as Shaman

...and much more!

Other Mandrake Titles:

Fries/*Cauldron of the Gods: a manual of Celtic Magick.*
552pp, royal octavo, 9781869928612 £24.99$40 paper

Fries/*Seidways Shaking, Swaying and Serpent Mysteries.* 350pp
9781869928360 £15/$25
Still the definitive and much sought after study of magical
trance and possession techniques.

Fries/*Helrunar - a manual of rune magick.* 454pp
9781968828902 pbk, £19.99/$40 Over 130 illustrations.
new enlarged and improved edition
'*...eminently practical and certainly breaks new ground.*' - Ronald
Hutton

Order direct from

Mandrake of Oxford

PO Box 250, Oxford, OX1 1AP (UK)

Phone: 01865 243671

(for credit card sales)

Prices include economy postage

Visit our web site

online at - www.mandrake.uk.net

Lightning Source UK Ltd.
Milton Keynes UK
UKOW07f0157151114

241641UK00001B/9/P